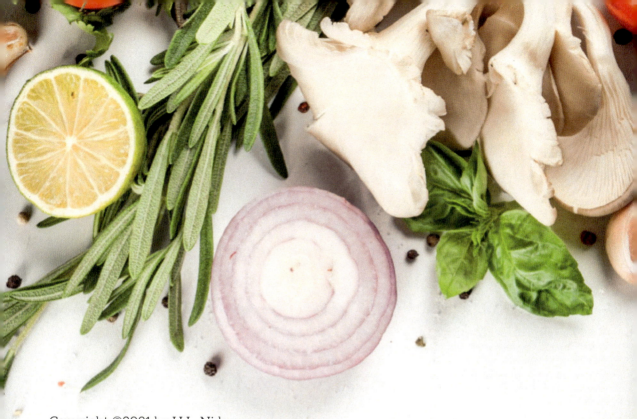

Copyright ©2021 by H.L. Nida

All Rights Reserved

No portion of this work may be reproduced in any format without written permission from the author and/or publisher, except as permitted by U.S. Copyright law. No part of this book may be stored in a retrieval system, transmitted in any form, by any means electronic, mechanical, photocopying, or recording, or otherwise, without express written permission from the author and/or publisher.

The recipes in this book were created in the authors kitchen from her personal knowledge of ingredients and years of experience. It is possible that another body of work has created recipes similar to those found in this book. If so, it is unintentional.

You know your health, if there's any question about ingredients in this cookbook or general compatibility with your personal situation, please consult your doctor. Author and publisher are not responsible for any adverse reaction or affects these recipes may have on someone with extreme allergies, or health conditions.

Published by Adin Publishing 2021
Edited by Adin Services & Bambi Sommers
Photography by Isabell Nida & Adin Services

ISBN: 978-1-7342274-9-9

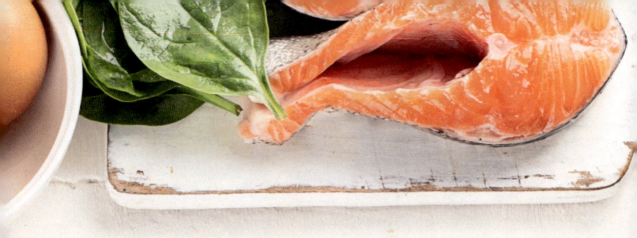

"Today, more than 95% of all chronic disease is caused by food choice, toxic food ingredients, nutritional deficiencies and lack of physical exercise."
— Mike Adams

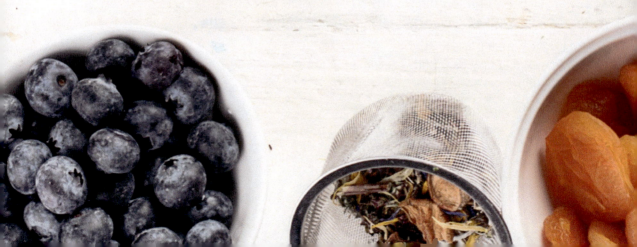

"Necessity is the mother of invention."

- English Proverb

My Story

Several years ago, I was diagnosed with multiple autoimmune diseases. Some were not a shock, as I knew family members to have similar issues, but others were a bit of a surprise. What was most shocking to me, was how my body had completely changed and how my quality of life started to slip away, a little more each day.

I was also surprised at how long it took to find a doctor that could diagnose me correctly. I went to various specialists and even tried Chinese medicine as well as Functional Wellness practitioners, which was an interesting as well as a very expensive experiment. There are many different types of doctors out there and they all treat their patients differently.

I went from being an active healthy adult to a couch potato in what seemed like 60 seconds flat! Even today, I cannot comprehend how quickly it happened and how my body transitioned from something I normally didn't have to think about, to something I had to force myself to use. It's a scary and crazy place to find yourself when your body doesn't respond normally to anything. Then when you find out that the food you consume is part of the problem, well that's when your life is turned upside down.

So, in my quest to figure out how to heal myself, I was put on an elimination diet. Which is awful, but worth the few weeks it takes to determine what your body can and cannot tolerate. After blood tests and other diagnostics, it's was determined that I'm a celiac (allergic to gluten). Well, okay that's not so horrible…. but I'm also allergic to soy, and my body doesn't tolerate dairy well, and I need to cut down on my inflammation, so that means no sugar or alcohol either. This was a shock to hear when I've lived what is considered a normal American diet my entire life. I thought I ate healthy! Boy was I surprised to find out what healthy eating really looks like, and the battle against food processing I was about to take.

What's even more shocking is when you start to read the labels of the items in your pantry! Did you know almost all chocolate has soy in it? Did you know that most condiments, salad dressings and sauces have added cane sugar, gluten or soy in them? Items that you would never expect to contain toxic and inflammatory ingredients – usually do. I remember when I had to clean my pantry out. I placed all the items I could no longer eat on my kitchen island. Then I looked at what I had left in the house that I am able to eat and I realized that about eighty percent of my pantry needed to be thrown away. That was a very frustrating day.

It felt like insanity to me! I was upset when I went to the store and looked at the cost of just one loaf of gluten free bread – but I couldn't buy it because it had sugar, soy, or dairy in it. I was feeling sick about 95% of the time at this point, and now I'm in a grocery store feeling helpless because I couldn't find food that I can eat. It was this moment when I realized that it was going to be an uphill battle to re-learn how to feed myself. Which seemed impossible as food is a basic human need that most of us don't need to think about. I was frustrated, no one else understood how tough this was and I felt extremely isolated.

For years now I've been experimenting with food, whole foods, foods that can and will help you feel better. Foods that even though you need to cook them yourself, as eating out is almost impossible now.

I hope these recipes will not only fill your stomach, but will help you feel better and become healthier.

"Food should be cleansing;
it should be restorative.
It should be fun."
— James Colquhoun, Food Matters

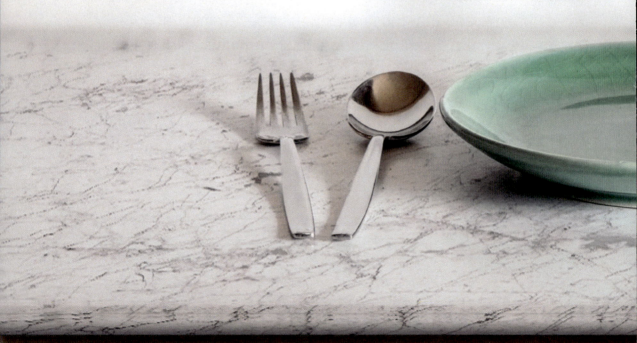

Organics are a Big Deal

I've spent a lot of time reading about the food we feed our bodies with and how it affects the entirety of our health. I have come to the conclusion that we need to consume organic products as much as possible, if possible, choose only organics. I have even decided to use shampoo, soap, cleaning supplies, almost everything in my life in an organic form. If I can find it as an organic product, that's how I buy it.

There's an amazing Ted Talk out there by a woman named Dr. Terry Wahls, a doctor of Neurology, who contracted Multiple Sclerosis and beat it! Surprisingly, not by how she was treating her patients with this very same disease, but because she decided to confront her wellness with what she knew was the main issue, her food! Give it a quick search, she has many, many videos out there about her health struggle and how she's made herself well from changing how she eats. Her number one recommendation is to eat organics!

Will eating healthy and organic be expensive? Yes! I can assure you that it will, but here's the bright side. You're taking control of your health! What is more expensive, food that will make your body whole, or more frequent visits to the doctor's office and paying for prescriptions?

Think about it this way, every cell within your body is fueled by what you consume. If you're consuming a large amount of processed foods filled with chemicals and toxins, when your cells regenerate, how healthy are they bound to be with this kind of fuel? Your nutritional intake is feeding every cell, every hair follicle, every skin cell, every organ, every corpuscle of blood your body makes. Do you want to tell your body you respect it, or not?

This is not a diet book, and I do not condone or approve of any of the diets or diet programs out there. In fact, I'm actually uninformed about the newest and best diets being offered, as I DO NOT DIET. I live a healthy lifestyle. This won't end after thirty days and I will somehow be "fixed." This is how I live. This is how I maintain my health, and how I'm trying to reverse the disease I have obviously participated in creating by my previous bad choices. This is self-care!

NOW LET'S DISCUSS GMO's!

The FDA has stated that GMO's (genetically modified organisms) are safe for us to consume. WHAT? Let me take a minute to explain a bit about GMO's.

A GMO is defined as any organism that has been altered using genetic engineering techniques, in a way that does not occur naturally. According to the USDA, GMO seeds are used in 90% of all corn, cotton and soy! NINETY PERCENT! GMO's trigger allergies and inflammation, as these seeds are specifically modified to not kill the crop from the insane amount of pesticides being sprayed on them. Think about that! In addition to that, once the food is modified it may have been altered with a wheat product. Well, if you're a celiac, that's a problem! And the worst part about all of this is that the USA has no requirement for food manufacturers to label a product as a GMO!

GMO's have been banned in Australia, France, Germany, Austria, Greece, Hungary, Japan, as well as the entire E.U., and the list goes on. So why does America, Canada and of course the inventor of this heinous idea China, allow GMO's into our food? I wish I knew!

In fact, in America while it's not a requirement for food manufacturers to label their products as GMO's, our government is regulating and fining Organic Farmers more than any other. Why?

The only way you can avoid GMO's is to only buy organic products. If it's organic isn't not a GMO. Some products label their items as NON-GMO, which is still better than eating products that don't tell you what's inside of them.

If you're purchasing fresh produce, here's a way to help read between the lines on the label. Each piece of produce should have a PLU number. If the number is four digits and is in the 3000'S or 4000's it has been conventionally produced – so it's full of chemicals and toxins. If the PLU is 5 digits and starts with a 9 it's organically grown produce. If the PLU is 5 digits and starts with an 8, IT'S A GMO!

READ YOUR LABELS!

Just because something says it's organic, doesn't mean it's good for you!

Be careful while grocery shopping! I do not recommend using a delivery service. I understand if you can't avoid it, but if you can, shop for yourself, because you need to read your labels!

Labels are deceiving. Make sure you read them thoroughly. Soy is in almost everything, including chocolate, gluten free breads and baked goods, mayonnaise, condiments, you name it, they'll put it in there. Why? Because it's cheap!

This also goes for sugar! Sugar has so many names the FDA allows food manufactures to substitute for it, that it's often hidden. Sometimes they hide it in the words "other natural flavors!" How this is legal?

When buying nut butters, make sure they only contain nuts and salt. No sugar or other ingredients.

When buying baking soda, make sure it's aluminum free.

When buying vanilla extract, don't buy it if it states it has any ingredient labeled as "other natural flavors." I only recommend Organic and PURE vanilla extract. Some manufacturers use a gland near a beaver's anus called castoreum to make vanilla flavoring! And, of course, the FDA says it's safe for us to consume!

My rule is, if I can't pronounce it, or I don't know what it is, I don't buy it! Also, if it has a TV commercial, you don't want it – except avocados – everyone wants avocados! Anytime a product says "low fat" or "sugar free" equate those phrases to the admission of chemicals and toxins in the food, because that's really what it's saying!

Shop smart, and if you can't find it, make it yourself from simple organic ingredients.

And finally, a friendly warning about choosing this lifestyle.

The most important thing that you will need in order to be successful at this lifestyle change is support from your loved ones. Your family, friends, roommates and of course any live-in boy/girlfriend can have a huge impact on how smoothly and successfully this change is for you.

A lot of people who don't have chronic health issues will make the most ridiculous claims - if you tell them what you're doing. Trust me, I've heard them all. I actually stopped being invited to do things with people because I do not drink alcohol and eat gluten! Yep, people are that shallow!

Buckle up, because this is a bumpy ride. It costs money and sometimes, it can cost a friend or two. But honestly, who wants a friend who isn't interested in your fight to reclaim your own health?

If I do end up in a social situation, I usually keep my mouth shut and have a water while engaging in social activity. Other times, I choose not to attend, as it can be overwhelming for me (I'm not a super social person to begin with). Figure out what works for you, but remember, not everyone will understand. And you need resign yourself to being okay with that.

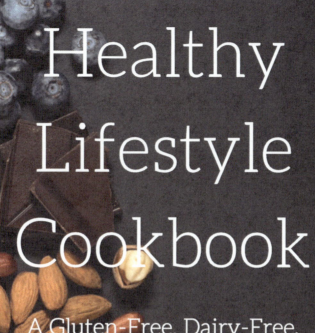

Healthy Lifestyle Cookbook

A Gluten-Free, Dairy-Free, Cane Sugar Free, Soy-Free Cookbook for anyone suffering from inflammation, auto immune diseases as well as other health issues.

H.L. Nida

"People are fed by the food industry, which pays no attention to health, and are treated by the health industry, which pays no attention to food."

— Wendell Berry

"One day I'd like to visit a doctor that asks me about my diet before asking me what prescriptions I take."
- H.L. Nida

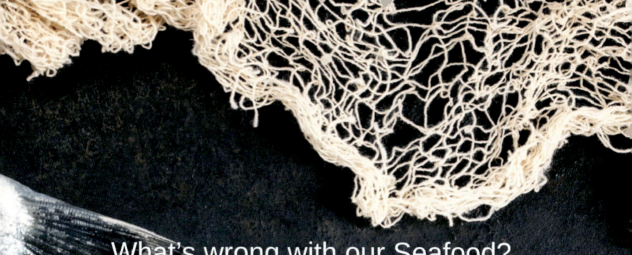

What's wrong with our Seafood?

Seafood is a great way to consume high quality protein with lots of essential fats that are very good for your health. Unfortunately, the seafood industry can be as deceiving as all the other food manufacturers.

We're all aware of imitation crab meat, because it's written on the label. But did you know that "wild caught" seafood might actually be farm raised? Or, that a lot of our seafood is imported from Asia? And don't even get me started on faux sea scallops!

For the purpose of this cookbook, I recommend wild caught seafood. But before we just check that it's written on the front of the package, let's dig a bit further to make sure we're paying for what we think we are. When you buy pre-packaged seafood, look to see if they have a website. It will help you to research how they fish and that they're not fishing "Wild Caught" fish from a net in the ocean. Yep, that's really happening. Farm Raised fish is typically not kept in clean living conditions, so the dirtier the fish's environment, the dirtier the fish is, and we don't want to eat that. I try to only purchase Salmon that is caught in Alaska. I like a few manufactures who not only tell you when the fish was caught, they'll tell you what river in Alaska they were caught in. Now that's transparency. If you're lucky enough to live near the ocean, I would purchase my fish from the fish markets at the boat docks. I lived in Florida and I think Grouper that's straight out of the Gulf of Mexico is the best damn dinner you'll ever have!

Be aware - sea scallops are not perfectly round, but they are always level. If one side is taller than the other or it's perfectly round, you're more than likely eating stingray meat.

Do your research, when you're not capable of purchasing your seafood fresh from the ocean, you need to know more than the package is telling you!

"Medicine is not healthcare.
Food is healthcare.
Medicine is sick care.
Let's all get this straight, for a change."

— Unknown

No Gluten, Diary, Soy, Cane Sugar, or Alcohol Included!

These ingredients are either a high allergen, or toxic to the human body.

Alcohol is poison, so is sugar. These two things are so toxic they are the main culprit for most of Americas illnesses. Diabetes 1 & 2, cancer, alcoholism, liver and kidney issues, brain fog, brain malfunctions, depression, anxiety...the list goes on! Did you know that cancer patients should not be given sugar, as cancer feeds on sugar, allowing cancer cells to rapidly multiply?

I remember being told as a kid during "Health" class to eat based on the government suggested food pyramid. I look at that food pyramid now and realize where I got my autoimmune issues! It's crazy what society will tell you is safe for you to consume, when government and big business rake in our cash, only to send us to the doctor who then ends up taking the rest of it.

Soy is junk food at its finest. There are so many articles out now, specifically if you're a vegan or vegetarian that will tote the wonders of the soy protein. Well, if it's so great, why is it so cheap? Think about that. Also, look at how many ways it is "processed." Obviously, this is not a healthy snack, and studies prove it causes inflammation. There are substitutes for soy if you look for them, but for some weird reason food manufacturers have put this ingredient in everything!

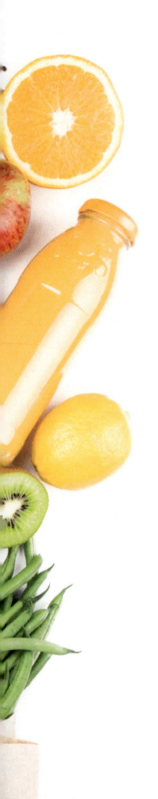

"The food you eat can
be either
the safest or most powerful
form of medicine,
or the slowest form of
poison"

— Ann Wigmore

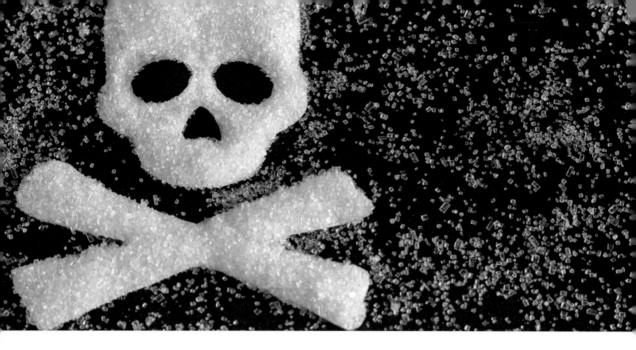

THE CURSE OF CANE SUGAR

In plain English, sugar is poison. I've made an effort to create recipes that still taste delicious without incorporating cane sugar. I've tried my very best to keep my sugar substitutions at or below 50 on the glycemic index. Cane sugar ranks at 100 on a scale from zero to one hundred. Here's where you will find the rankings of the three sugar replacements I use in this cookbook:

Organic Raw Honey	30*
Organic Coconut Palm Sugar	35
Organic Maple Syrup	55

*If you're using processed honey, and not raw honey this will move your honey to the rank of 50.

Other names used for Sugar (not all inclusive): Fructose, Dextrose, Maltose, Saccharose, Sucrose, Erythritol, Syrup, Cane Juice, Glucose, Crystalline Fructose.

Food Manufacturers are so sneaky. They try to hide cane sugar behind these synonyms.

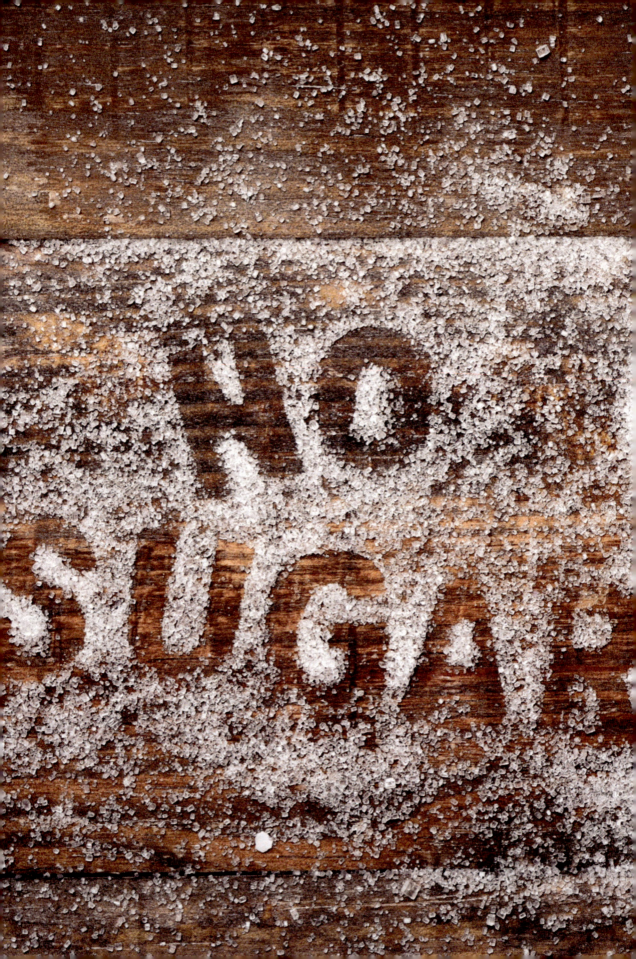

"Sugar is eight times as addictive as cocaine. And what's interesting is while cocaine and heroine activate only one spot for pleasure in the brain, sugar lights up the brain like a pinball machine."
— Dr. Mark Hyman

"Sugar is the most dangerous drug of the times and can still easily be acquired everywhere."
— Paul van der Velpen
— Head of Amsterdam's Health Service

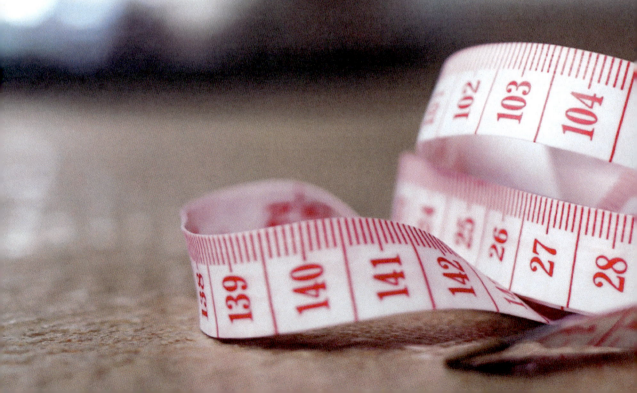

"Many people might not realize that the fat on their bodies actually, comes from the sugar they eat, not from the fat they eat."

—Dr. Berg

Coconut Oil vs. Palm Shortening

Here are some differences you might want to know about these oils before you start cooking these recipes.

First off, make sure if you are using Coconut Oil, that it's organic, AND refined. If not, everything will taste like coconut.

Palm Shortening is always a substitute for Coconut Oil, but Coconut Oil is not always a substitute for Palm Shortening. Personally, I prefer Palm Shortening to bake with. It makes baked goods less greasy. Coconut oil has a tendency to be greasy.

I know a lot of people who hate the taste of coconut, so if that's you, use Palm Shortening instead. There's no added flavor to Palm Shortening, so the recipes will work just as well with Palm Shortening as they do with Coconut Oil.

Palm Shortening has a lot of "bad" publicity associated with it. There are a lot of claims that the harvesting of this oil is destroying the rain forest. I have no first-hand knowledge of this, but I do try to purchase Responsibly or Certified Sustainable Organic Palm Shortening. Red Palm Shortening works just as well as others. There's no cholesterol associated with this product, it's free of trans fat carbs and is a natural source of antioxidants due to its richness in Vitamin E and Omega 6. So, for me, it's a win-win. Choose your favorite and stick with it or give them both equal time at your table. Either way you can't go wrong.

"There are way too many people counting calories and not enough counting chemicals."
— Unknown

Authors Notes

Before we get to my recipes, I want to provide you with full disclosure. I don't make these recipes every day.

The best way to maintain my health is to eat simply. I typically consume grilled meats minimally seasoned, with lots of vegetables for sides and fruit for dessert.

I use the recipes in this cookbook for special occasions, holidays, or for when I get bored with the simplicity of my diet. I do make a smoothie every day for breakfast or lunch, but breads and cookies are a delicacy that honestly, I don't want to live without because I have health issues.

I also lift weights and perform cardio at least three times a week to keep myself healthy and sane. If you're not working out, I highly suggest you get to a gym, buy the membership and start!

I hope you enjoy these recipes and I pray they make you feel comforted and satisfied, all while making better food decisions for a healthier life.

Enjoy!

"Want to be healthy?
COOK.
The food industry had done a great job of convincing eaters that corporations can cook better than we can.

The problem is, it's not true."

— Michael Pollan

CONTENTS:

Sauces, Condiments, Dips & Spices

Appetizers

Salads

Sides

Entrée's

Soups

Breakfast

Breads

Smoothies

Desserts

Cookies

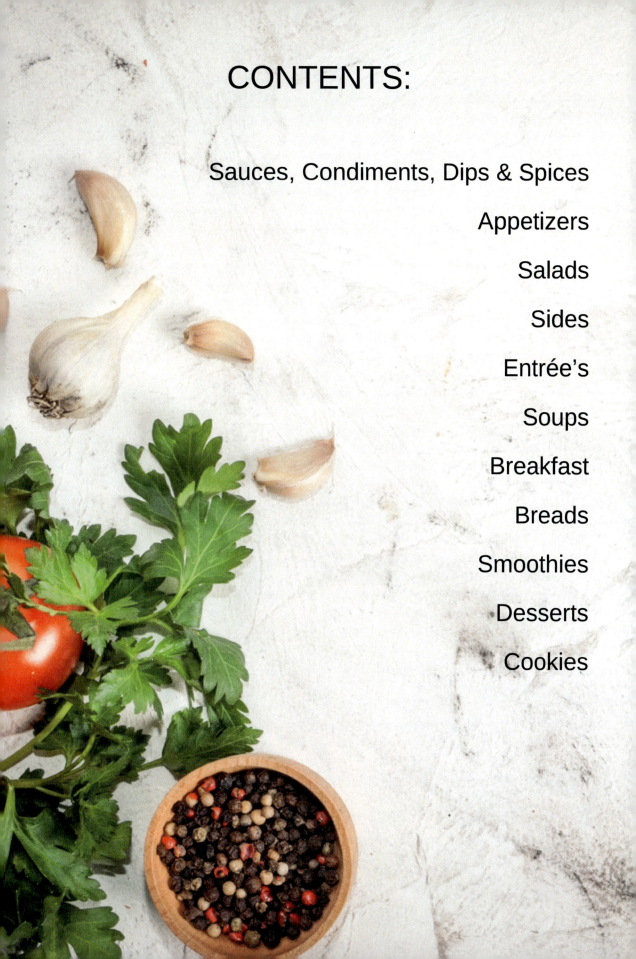

Sauces, Condiments, Dips & Spices

From top clockwise:
Ketchup - Page 29
Ranch Dressing - Page 32
Thousand Island Dressing - Page 33
Honey Mustard - Page 34

Ketchup

6 oz	Organic Tomato Paste
1-2 TBSP	Organic Apple Cider Vinegar
1 tsp	Organic Garlic Powder
1/8 tsp	Organic Dried Paprika
1/8 tsp	Organic Dried Turmeric
	Fresh Ground Salt & Pepper to taste
2-4 TBSP	Filtered or Purified Water

Mix all ingredients until well combined. Store in air-tight container inside of refrigerator.

If your ketchup is too thick, just add additional water until your desired thickness.

Pictured on Page 28 - top center - Photo by Isabell Nida

Mayonnaise

2 TBSP	Organic Lemon Juice
2 tsp	Organic Apple Cider Vinegar
2	Organic Egg Yolks
1 tsp	Organic Raw Honey
1 tsp	Organic Ground Mustard
1/2 tsp	Sea Salt
1 C	Organic Safflower Oil
1 C	Organic Canola Oil

Mix all ingredients except oils in a food processor on medium speed to combine. Open top, leaving on medium speed and add oil very slowly with the processor running. This should take between 3 to 5 minutes to add the oils – so be patient. In 1 -2 minutes you should observe the oils thickening.

Store in an airtight container with a large opening in your refrigerator for 1 – 2 weeks.

You can substitute oils listed with Avocado Oil, Extra Virgin Olive Oil or any oil that you like the taste of. Make sure your oil choice is high-quality and of course, that it's organic.

Tzatziki Sauce

1 C	Organic Dairy-Free Unsweetened Yogurt
1	Organic Cucumber
3 cloves	Organic Garlic
1 TBSP	Organic Apple Cider Vinegar
1 1/2 TBSP	Organic Virgin Olive Oil
1/2 TBSP	Organic Dried Dill Weed
	Fresh Ground Salt and Pepper to taste

Cut ends and partial skin off of the cucumber. Using a cheese grater, grate the entire cucumber. Place grated cucumber inside a paper towel (or several) and squeeze excess water from cucumber.

Combine yogurt, grated cucumber, pressed garlic and additional ingredients thoroughly. Place in air-tight container and chill for at least six hours before serving. It tastes best the next day if you have time to make beforehand.

Ranch Dressing

1/3 C	Mayonnaise – Page 30
1/3 C	Organic Non-Dairy Unsweetened Yogurt
1 TBSP	Organic Sweet Onion - grated
1 tsp	Organic Dried Chives
1 tsp	Organic Dried Dill Weed
1/4 tsp	Organic Garlic Powder
1/4 tsp	Organic Dried Basil
	Fresh Ground Salt & Pepper to taste

Combine all ingredients and store in air-tight container in your refrigerator.

This will only last as long as the earliest date on either your yogurt or mayonnaise (as stated, so be mindful when making with ingredients that are about to expire.

If you want to make it thicker and more like a dip, use more mayonnaise than almond yogurt and keep the rest of the ingredients the same. I do this when I make my chicken wings, so the ranch sticks to them better, or when using as a veggie dip.

Pictured on Page 28 - left - Photo by Isabell Nida

Thousand Island Dressing

1/2 C	Organic Mayonnaise – Page 30
3 TBSP	Organic Ketchup - Page 29
2 TBSP	Organic Pickle Relish - no sugar added
1 TBSP	Organic Apple Cider Vinegar
1 TBSP	Organic Raw Honey
	Fresh ground Salt and Pepper to taste

Combine all ingredients and store in an air-tight container in your refrigerator.

I confess, this is not my favorite dressing, but it is my husband's favorite, and once I started reading the labels of the brands available at the grocery store, I had to come up with a healthy alternative for him. So, if you like Thousand Island, you can thank my husband for this recipe!

Honey Mustard Dressing/Dip

3/4 C   Organic Mayonnaise – Page 30
1/2 C   Organic Spicy, Dijon or Yellow Mustard
2 TBSP   Organic Raw Honey

Combine all ingredients and store in an air-tight container in your refrigerator.

You can add ¼ tsp of parsley, or fresh ground salt and pepper if you'd like to add some visual appeal as well as a slightly more refined taste. In my home, the hubby doesn't always appreciate my variances, but maybe you will.

Serves well as a salad dressing. It's also a great dip for sweet potato fries or grilled chicken.

Pictured on Page 28 - left - Photo by Isabell Nida

Mango Sauce

1	Organic Ripe Mango - cut into pieces
1	Organic Jalapeno
1 TBSP	Organic Lime Juice
1-2 Cloves	Fresh Organic Garlic
	Fresh Ground salt and pepper to taste

In blender or food processor, blend all ingredients on mix until combined. If you're a spicy person, add more jalapeno or only use ½ of a jalapeno if spice is an issue for you.

Keep in an air-tight container in the fridge, should last about a week or maybe more.

This sauce is great on rice, fish, or chicken.

Pineapple Sauce

1/4	Fresh Organic Pineapple - cut in chunks
1/2	Organic Yellow Bell Pepper
1	Organic Clove Garlic - slightly chopped
1 TBSP	Organic Avocado Oil
1/2 tsp	Organic Dried Cilantro
1/4 tsp	Organic Dried Cayenne Pepper
	Fresh Ground Salt and Pepper to taste

In blender or food processor, blend all ingredients on high until combined. If you're a spicy person, add more Jalapenos or only use ½ of a jalapeno if spice is an issue for you.

Store in fridge in an air-tight container.

This is my favorite sauce for fish and shellfish. It has a spicy sweet taste and when I'm not on vacation, it makes me feel like I am.

Pizza Sauce

6 oz	Organic Tomato Paste
1/4 C	Purified Water
1/2 tsp	Organic Onion Powder
1/2 tsp	Organic Garlic Powder
1 tsp	Organic Dried Oregano
1 tsp	Organic Dried Basil
1/4 tsp	Organic Dried Thyme
	Fresh Ground Salt and Pepper to taste

Mix all ingredients in small bowl. Makes just enough sauce for my 18" pizza dough recipe – Page 138.

I know this recipe is beyond simple, but it's actually very good and super quick to make. It leaves space for your toppings to still tickle your taste buds.

B-B-Q Sauce

1	Organic Medium Onion - chopped
3 cloves	Organic Garlic - minced
3 TBSP	Organic Coconut Oil
1 C	Organic Pitted Dates
2 C	Organic Pitted Cherries
1 TBSP	Smoked Sea Salt
1 TBSP	Liquid Smoke
2 TBSP	Organic White Balsamic Vinegar
1 TBSP	Organic Maple Syrup or Raw Honey*
	Fresh Ground Salt & Pepper to taste

Sauté onions and garlic in oil until translucent and aromatic in large pan or skillet.

Add remaining ingredients and simmer over low heat for 20–25 minutes, stirring often. It will be ready when the ingredients have cooked down and thickened in the pan, it should coat your spoon. Make sure not to cook off all the fluids, as this will make your sauce very thick.

Remove from heat and put into a blender or food processor. Mix thoroughly until it reaches the consistency of sauce. To make this sugar free, I use unsweetened blackberry vinegar instead of maple syrup or honey and it tastes amazing!

Tartar Sauce

1/2 C	Organic Mayonnaise – Page 30
1 TBSP	Organic Lemon Juice
3 TBSP	Organic Dill Pickles
2 TBSP	Organic Onion
1/2 TBSP	Organic Dried Dill Weed
	Fresh Ground Salt and Pepper to taste

In a small mixing bowl, combine the mayonnaise and lemon juice. Mince onions. Dry dill pickles with cloth or paper towel and lightly squeeze out excess moisture, then mince into tiny pieces. Add onion, pickle and spices to mayonnaise mixture and leave overnight in refrigerator before serving.

Store in airtight container in your refrigerator.

Cocktail Sauce

1/2 C	Organic Ketchup – Page 29
2 TBSP	Organic Horseradish Root

Combine ingredients thoroughly. Store in air-tight container.

Only use horseradish root, usually found in the refrigerated section of your grocery store. It should only have one ingredient – horseradish! Do not use prepared horseradish, as it always comes with inflammatory ingredients added and the taste will be altered significantly. You can always add more or less depending on how hot you want your cocktail sauce to taste.

If you're a die-hard horseradish lover, grate your own from a fresh root to use.

Nut Butter Fruit Dip

1/2 C   Organic Nut Butter - your choice
1/4 C   Organic Unsweetened Non-Dairy Yogurt
2 TBSP   Organic Raw Honey

Combine ingredients thoroughly and serve immediately.

This will keep if stored in an airtight container in your refrigerator for as long as the expiration date on your yogurt.

Tastes great with sliced apples or bananas.

You can substitute any nut butter, if you prefer one over another.

Pictured on Page 42 - left - Photo by Isabell Nida

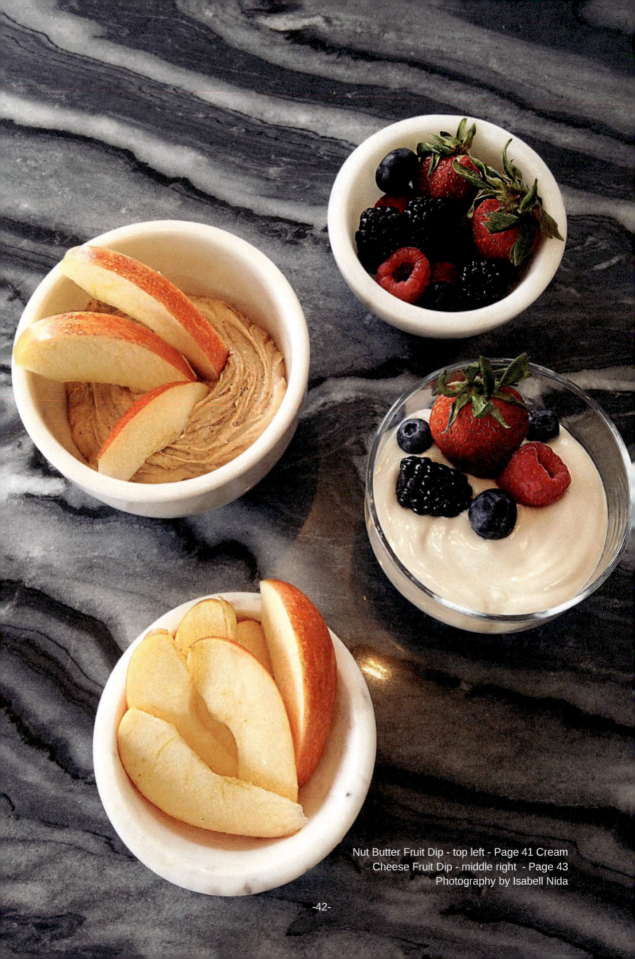

Nut Butter Fruit Dip - top left - Page 41 Cream Cheese Fruit Dip - middle right - Page 43
Photography by Isabell Nida

Cream Cheese Fruit Dip

1/4 C	Organic Plain Dairy-Free Cream Cheese
1/4 C	Organic Dairy-Free Unsweetened Yogurt
1 – 3 TBSP	Organic Raw Honey
1/4 tsp	Organic Vanilla Extract

Combine all ingredients until smooth. Serve immediately with your fruit of choice.

This will keep if stored in an airtight container in your refrigerator for as long as the expiration date on your yogurt.

This is fabulous with berries, bananas, even tropical fruit. It's always a huge hit as an appetizer or dessert at dinner parties.

Pictured on Page 42 - Photo by Isabell Nida

Jerk Spice

1 tsp	Organic Garlic Powder
1 tsp	Organic Cayenne Pepper
1 tsp	Organic Paprika
1 tsp	Organic Allspice
1 tsp	Organic Thyme
1 tsp	Organic Parsley
1/2 tsp	Organic Cumin
1/2 tsp	Organic Cloves
1/2 tsp	Organic Cinnamon
1/2 tsp	Sea Salt
1/2 tsp	Organic Ground Pepper

Combine in small mixing bowl.

I save my old glass spice jars, peel off the labels and wash them in the dishwasher to use for my own spice combinations. If you really want a large amount of this spice, use same amounts in tablespoons instead of teaspoons, it'll fill up a jar and a half.

Mediterranean Spice

2 TBSP	Sea Salt
1 TBSP	Organic Lemon Zest
2 tsp	Organic Garlic Powder
1 tsp	Organic Red Pepper
1 tsp	Organic Oregano
1 tsp	Organic Ground Pepper

Combine in small mixing bowl. Store in an air-tight container.

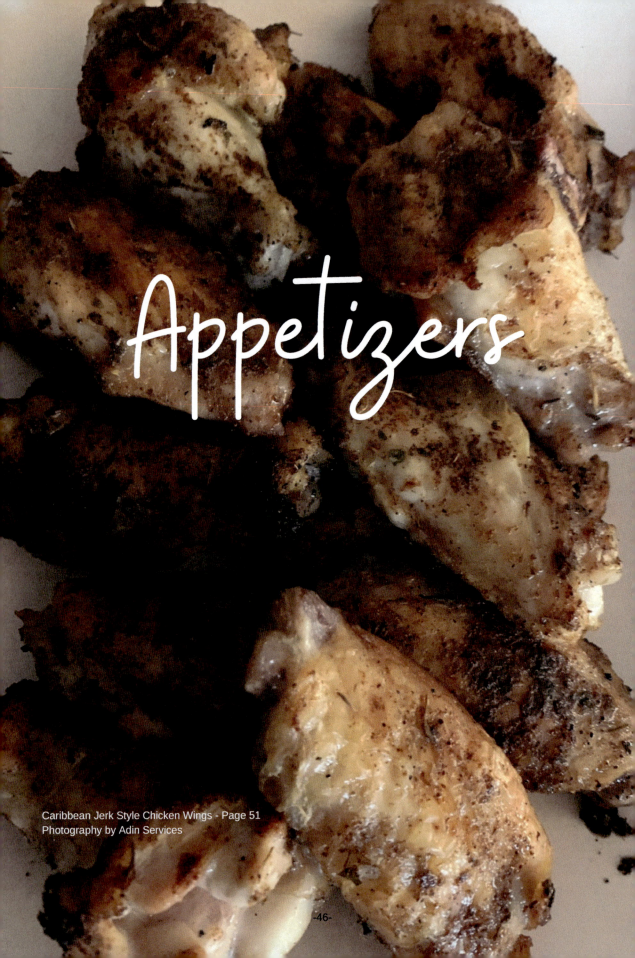

Caribbean Jerk Style Chicken Wings - Page 51
Photography by Adin Services

Scallop Appetizer

20	Wild Caught Medium Sized Sea Scallops
2 TBSP	Organic Margarine
3 TBSP	Organic Onion - minced
4 oz	Organic White Mushrooms - sliced thin
	Fresh Ground Salt & Pepper to taste
1/4 C	Organic Chicken or Veggie Broth
1/4 C	Organic Unsweetened Non-Dairy Cream
1	Organic Egg Yolk
1/4 tsp	Organic Cayenne Pepper
1/2 tsp	Organic Chives
1 tsp	Organic Lemon zest

On the stove top in a skillet, melt margarine on medium heat. When melted add onions and sliced mushrooms to sauté. Sprinkle with salt and pepper. Add broth and heat until simmering.

Poach scallops in broth vegetable mixture for approximately 2 minutes each side. Then place scallops, mushrooms and onions on small dishes separately and set aside – keep warm.

Scallop Appetizer - Continued

Add non-dairy cream to strained broth and turn heat to high. Simmer on high until it reduces by half and thickens. When it's thickened, a spatula run across the bottom of pan will make a line that lasts about 30 seconds. Turn off heat and let sit one minute. Whisk in egg yolk very quickly. Add spices and zest as you continue to whisk. Set aside.

In ramekins or scallop shells (if you have them) layer the onions and mushrooms on the bottom, place 5 scallops in each, then cover with sauce.

Place ramekins inside baking dish that can hold all four at once and broil about 10 inches below heat, for 5-10 minutes.

Serve immediately.

Buffalo Chicken Wings

2 lb	Organic Chicken Wings
3/4 C	Organic Cassava Flour
1/4 C	Organic Arrowroot Flour
1/4 tsp	Organic Garlic Powder
1/2 tsp	Organic Mustard Powder
1 tsp	Organic Dried Chives
1/2-1 tsp	Organic Cayenne Pepper
	Fresh Ground Salt and pepper to taste
1/2 C	Organic Coconut Oil
1/4 C	Organic Margarine - melted
1/3 C	Organic Hot Sauce

Mix all dry ingredients together in a large bowl. Place chicken wings in dry ingredients and coat (I use my hands to ensure they're coated well).

Heat coconut oil in large enamel skillet, on medium setting (avoid letting the oil get too hot). Place coated chicken wings carefully in oil. Cook until 165 degrees internally; chicken should be light brown. Flip several times while frying. If your oil starts to run low you can add more.

Buffalo Chicken Wings - continued

Once wings are cooked thoroughly place on wire rack with paper towel on top to let cool.

Melt margarine in large bowl (big enough to hold all of your wings). Add hot sauce and whisk. Place cooked wings into the bowl and swirl until wings are coated.

Serve wings with ranch dressing and celery sticks.

Caribbean Jerk Style Chicken Wings
Baked or Grilled

2 lb   Organic Chicken Wings
1 C   Organic Coconut Oil

1/3 C   Jerk Spice - Page 39

The night before (if possible rinse and pat dry your chicken wings. Place in large bowl with a tight lid. Add in 1/3 C Jerk Seasoning and shake to ensure all wings are covered with seasoning.Place in refrigerator overnight to let the spices sink into the meat. Feel free to actually rub the spices in with your hands if you prefer.

Place in preheated 400-degree oven for 20 minutes, turning at halfway. If your wings are extra-large you may need to bake longer.

If you choose to grill, grill on top of a grill mat for at least 10 minutes each side, keeping in mind if your cooking large wings you may need more time to grill.

Serve wings with ranch dressing and celery sticks.

Pictured on Page 46 Photo by Adin Services

Guacamole

2 large	Ripe Organic Avocados
1/4 C	Organic Onion – chopped
1/4 C	Fresh Organic Cilantro - chopped
1	Organic Lime - squeezed
	Fresh Ground Salt and Pepper to taste

Chop up avocados and place inside of a medium sized bowl. Add chopped onion, cilantro and squeezed lime and crush with the tines of a fork, keeping it slightly chunky. Add salt and pepper to taste.

You can add chopped organic tomatoes, organic garlic, or chopped jalapeno peppers to add additional spice or flavor.

This stuff is addicting, so you've been warned. Obviously, it goes great with chips, on top of hamburgers or Mexican food, but I like it on almost anything, but that's because I'm already addicted!

Pictured on Page 90 - Photography by Adin Services

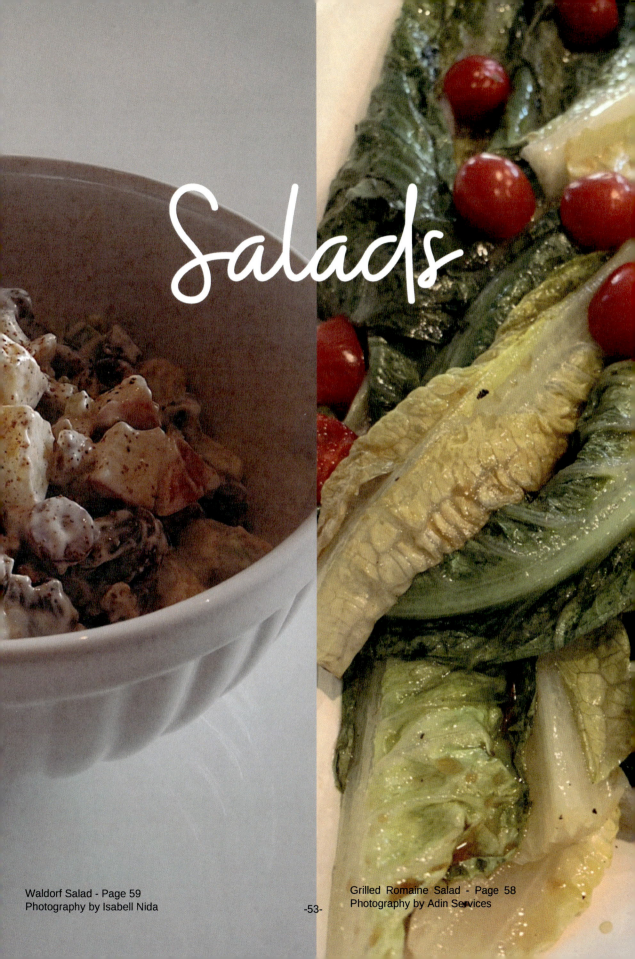

Salads

Waldorf Salad - Page 59
Photography by Isabell Nida

Grilled Romaine Salad - Page 58
Photography by Adin Services

Chicken Salad

2 C	Organic Chicken Breast - precooked Organic
1/2 C	Mayonnaise – Page 30
2 TBSP	Organic Spicy Mustard
1/4 C	Organic Chopped Sweet Onion
3 stalks	Organic Celery - chopped
1/3 C	Organic Unsweetened Cranberries - chopped
1 TBSP	Lemon White Balsamic Vinegar
1 TBSP	Organic Dried Parsley
1 TBSP	Organic Dried Coriander
1/2 TBSP	Fresh Organic Lemon Juice
	Fresh Ground Salt and Pepper to taste

Shred or chop precooked chicken into small pieces.

Combine all ingredients in a large bowl, ensuring they are mixed thoroughly.

Serve on large tray lined with lettuce.

Tastes great on bread for a sandwich, with almond crackers or just get a fork and eat it right out of the bowl. Delicious!

Baked Potato Salad

This is one recipe I've never shared. No matter how many times I've been asked. I guess now everyone will know my secret to making the best potato salad ever!

6 large	Organic Russet Potatoes
3	Organic Boiled Eggs
1 large	Organic Sweet Onion
2/3 C	Organic Mayonnaise – Page 30
1/4 C	Organic Mustard - I prefer Spicy Brown
1 TBSP	Organic Apple Cider Vinegar
1 TBSP	Organic Chopped Chives
1 TBSP	Organic Chopped Parsley
1 1/2 tsp	Organic Celery Seed or Celery Salt
	Fresh Ground Salt and Pepper to taste

Cut off ends and skin of onion, place inside a large square of foil and put with foil wrapped Potatoes in oven at 450 degrees until potatoes are soft (usually 1 ½ to 2 hours).

While potatoes are baking, prepare the dressing by combining all ingredients from mayonnaise to salt and pepper together in a large bowl, stir well to combine. Chop up boiled eggs into small pieces, add to dressing.

Baked Potato Salad - Continued

When potatoes and onion are cooked, place onions and any juices in the foil into a medium sized bowl. Use two knives to slice through the onion until it's very finely chopped. You don't want it to be so finely chopped that there aren't any chunks of onion left, but it should be mostly mushy. Add onions to dressing.

When potatoes are cool, cut each in half, length wise. Use a spoon to scoop out the insides of the potatoes directly into the dressing. Combine and serve either warm or cold.

Sweet Potato Salad

3 large	Organic Sweet Potatoes
1/2	Organic Onion
2 TBSP	Organic Avocado Oil
4	Pre-Baked No Nitrate Turkey Bacon
1/2 C	Organic Mayonnaise – Page 30
1 1/2 TBSP	Organic Horseradish Root - not prepared
1 tsp	Organic Dried Coriander
1 tsp	Smoked Sea Salt
1/2 tsp	Organic Dried Basil
	Fresh Ground Black Pepper to taste

Preheat oven to 425 degrees.

Peel and chop sweet potatoes into small pieces. Peel and slice onion vertically. Place both in a large mixing bowl and toss with avocado oil, coat evenly. Place onto baking sheet and roast for 25 – 30 minutes. Onions should brown slightly and sweet potatoes should be thoroughly baked.

Remove from oven and let cool. In mixing bowl combine ingredients from mayonnaise through ground pepper. Crumble in pre-cooked bacon, then add cooled potato and onion mixture. Serve warm, or cold. This is a great savory side dish that compliments chicken meals well.

Grilled Romaine Salad

2 heads	Organic Romaine Lettuce
1/4 C	Organic Olive Oil
1/2 small	Organic Onion
4 oz	Organic Mushrooms
2 TBSP	Lemon White Balsamic Vinegar
	Fresh Ground Salt and Pepper to taste

Wash and clean romaine lettuce after detaching from stalk. Slice half of a small onion in very thin slices. Slice mushrooms thinly as well.

Place lettuce on grill mat and sprinkle with olive oil, coating both sides of each leaf. This is not an exact science, so don't OCD about it. Add sliced mushrooms and onions and toss with vinegar. Add salt and pepper and place grill mat on hot preheated grill.

Stay at the grill and turn lettuce and veggies as it cooks. Be careful, the oil will make some flames flash. Cook until wilted. Serve immediately.

This dish is simple, but it's delicious!

Pictured on Page 53- Photography by Adin Services
Pictured on Page 79 - Photography by Isabell Nida

Waldorf Salad

4 medium	Organic Apples - your choice
1 TBSP	Organic Lemon Juice
1/2 C	Organic Celery - chopped
1/2 C	Organic Seedless Grapes - halved
1/2 C	Walnuts - chopped
1/3 C	Organic Raisins
1/2 C	Organic Mayonnaise – Page 30
1 TBSP	Organic Raw Honey
1/2 tsp	Organic Lemon Juice
1/2 C	Organic Dairy Free Unsweetened Yogurt
dash	Organic Ground Nutmeg

Dice apples with skin on, place in a large mixing bowl and sprinkle with the tablespoon lemon juice. Add in celery, grapes, walnuts and raisins and stir to combine.

In a small mixing bowl combine mayonnaise, honey, lemon juice and yogurt. Pour over apples and fold until combined. Chill immediately until ready to serve. Keep in refrigerator in air-tight container.

Sprinkle nutmeg on top before serving.

Pictured on Page 53 - Photography by Isabell Nida

SIDES

Sweet Potato Fries - Page 64
Honey Mustard Dip - Page 34
Photography by Adin Services

Home Made French Fries

1 – 2 lbs   Organic Russet Potatoes
1/3 C   Organic Coconut Oil
               Freshly Ground Sea Salt

In a 400-degree oven, bake foil wrapped potatoes for 45 minutes to an hour depending on the size of your potatoes. When done, they should not be fully baked. Let cool.

Peel the skin off your pre-baked potatoes, or leave on if you prefer, and cut into desired length and width.

Heat oil in deep skillet on medium heat. When the oil is hot, lower a few pieces of potato at a time into skillet using tongs. When skillet is full without any overlapping pieces, fry until brown. Once browned, flip and brown the other side. When done, place on wire rack lined with paper towels. Keep adding potatoes to oil until all are cooked.

Add salt to taste and serve warm.

Use Honey Mustard Dip– Page 34 , Ketchup – Page 29, or Ranch Dressing - Page 32, to dip them in. Yummy!

Scalloped Potatoes

2 lbs	Organic Russet Potatoes - pre-baked
1/4 C	Organic Onion - grated
3 TBSP	Organic Margarine
2 1/2 TBSP	Organic Arrowroot Flour
1/4 tsp	Organic Ground Mustard
dash	Organic Cayenne Pepper
1 C	Organic Unsweetened Non-Dairy Milk
1/2 C	Organic Non-Dairy Half & Half or Cream
4 oz	Organic Non-Dairy Cream Cheese
1/2 C	Organic Non-Dairy Shredded Cheese

Pre-bake potatoes in oven at 400 degrees for an hour, to an hour and a half, depending on the size of your potatoes. Do not bake until fully cooked. Place in refrigerator overnight to cool, this makes them easier to slice. If you've forgotten to pre-bake the potatoes, place in pressure cooker on rack with 1 C water on bottom for 20 minutes and cool thoroughly before slicing.

On stovetop on medium heat melt the margarine in a saucepan. Add arrowroot flour and spices and whisk until bubbly. Then, pour in milk slowly and whisk until combined, add half and half.

Scalloped Potatoes - Continued

Finally add in the cream cheese and onions and continue to stir until thick and well combined.

Slice potatoes thinly, I like to use a food processor or a slicer to get them the same thickness.

Oil bottom and sides of a 9 x 9 baking dish. Layer the potato slices and sauce, until the dish is full, reserving sauce for the top. Pour remaining sauce on the top. You can add your favorite non-dairy shredded cheese to the top - optional.

Bake at 350 degrees for 30-40 minutes. The top should brown and the sauce should be bubbly. Serve warm. Store leftovers in air-tight container in refrigerator for up to 5 days.

Sweet Potato Fries

3 large   Organic Sweet Potatoes
1 C   Organic Coconut Oil
             Freshly Ground Sea Salt

Peel and cut sweet potatoes into desired sized pieces. If you've rinsed your potatoes after peeling, make sure to dry them off with a paper towel, to prevent the oil from splattering.

Place oil into a deep pan/skillet and heat on medium to low heat. Once oil is hot, drop in potatoes slowly, a few at a time with tongs, and heat through. I like to make sure they start to brown before turning. Only turn once.

You may have to exchange batches several times. Cool on wire rack with paper towel over it. Add freshly ground salt to taste.

Dip in Honey Mustard sauce – Page 34. Delicious and healthy!

Pictured on Page 60 - Photography by Adin Services

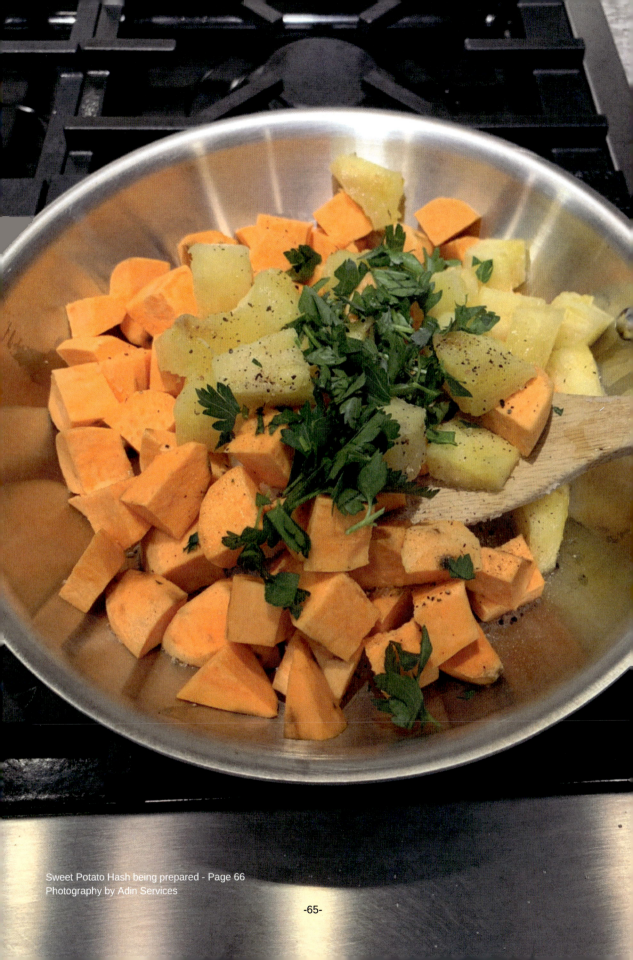

Sweet Potato Hash being prepared - Page 66
Photography by Adin Services

Sweet Potato Hash

3 large   Organic Sweet Potatoes
1/2   Fresh Organic Pineapple
1/4 C   Organic Coconut Oil
1 TBSP   Organic Parsley
            Fresh Ground Salt and Pepper to taste

Peel and cut sweet potatoes into bite-sized pieces, about 1 inch. Cut half your pineapple into small pieces. You should have more sweet potatoes than pineapple.

In large deep skillet, melt coconut oil. Place potatoes and pineapple in skillet together. Stir while cooking to ensure all pieces are cooked evenly. Sprinkle with parsley and salt and pepper and cook until the potatoes start to brown slightly and are soft when pierced with a fork.

Serve warm.

Pictured on Page 65 Photography by Adin Services

Sweet Potato Casserole

5-6	Organic Sweet Potatoes
1/2 C	Organic Orange Juice
1/4 C	Organic Coconut Palm Sugar
1/4 C	Organic Margarine - melted
1 TBSP	Organic Ground Cinnamon
1 tsp	Organic Ground Ginger
1/2 tsp	Organic Ground Nutmeg
1/2 tsp	Organic Ground Cloves

Topping:

1/4 C	Organic Almond Flour
1/2 C	Raw Pecans – chopped
3 TBSP	Organic Coconut Palm Sugar
1 tsp	Organic Cinnamon
3 TBSP	Organic Coconut Oil or Margarine

Bake sweet potatoes in foil at 400 degrees for about an hour to 1 ¼ hours. Timing will vary by the size of your potatoes. They will squish with your hand (inside a pot holder) when done. Let them cool enough to handle safely.

Sweet Potato Casserole - Continued

When cool, remove skin and place in large standing mixer. Add in orange juice, spices, melted margarine and coconut palm sugar. Mix on medium speed until well combined. Place inside a medium sized casserole dish.

To make topping, combine all ingredients in a medium sized bowl and use a pastry cutter to mix, ensuring the oil or margarine is thoroughly combined and evenly spread through the mixture. It should be crumbly in texture. Sprinkle on top of prepared potatoes.

Bake in oven at 350 degrees for 30-40 minutes, until heated through. If needed, cover with foil to ensure the topping does not burn.

Mashed Cauliflower

1 large   Organic Cauliflower Head
1/4 C   Organic Margarine
1 TBSP   Organic Dried Chives
              Fresh Ground Salt and Pepper to taste

In a large pot, boil entire head of cauliflower (cut to fit if needed). Boil continuously for 15 – 20 minutes until it is very soft, a fork should be able to be inserted into it without resistance.

Drain well, place cooked cauliflower in standing mixer, add additional ingredients and with paddle attachment mix on medium for 5 minutes.

Serve as a side dish to your favorite meal. You can top with gravy or sauce if desired.

Roasted Broccolini

1 lb	Organic Broccolini
	Organic Olive Oil
2 cloves	Organic Garlic
1 TBSP	Organic Lemon Zest
1 TBSP	Organic Parsley
	Fresh Ground Salt and Pepper to taste

Preheat oven to 350 degrees.

In a large casserole dish, place washed and dried broccolini so that the stalks are not touching. Drizzle broccolini with olive oil, be as stingy or as generous as you like. Sprinkle lemon zest, parsley and salt and pepper on top.

Place in middle rack of preheated oven for 30 – 35 minutes. When a fork can be inserted and removed easily, it's done.

Spiraled Veggies

1	Organic Zucchini - large
2	Organic Carrots - large
1-2 cloves	Organic Garlic
3 TBSP	Organic Olive Oil
1/2 tsp	Organic Dried Parsley
	Fresh Ground Salt & Pepper to taste

Spiral the zucchini and carrots and place into a medium sized mixing bowl.

Mince or smash garlic, ensuring no large chunks are left.

On stovetop in large saucepan or skillet, heat oil and add in smashed garlic. Stir to break up garlic into oil for a minute, then add spiraled vegetables and seasoning. Cook until desired tenderness, usually only about 5 minutes, stirring often. Add more oil if necessary.

Simple and delicious side dish that goes with almost any meal.

Get creative and add in some yucca root, sweet potato or cassava root. Anything you can spiral will work with this recipe.

Pictured on Page 90 Photo by Adin Services

Sauteed Mushrooms & Onions

8 oz	Organic Mushrooms - any type
1 small	Organic Onion
3 TBSP	Organic Margarine or Olive Oil
1 tsp	Organic Garlic – fresh or dried
1 TBSP	Organic Chives

Slice mushrooms and onions thinly. Mince garlic if you're using fresh.

In skillet on stove top heat margarine until melted. Add mushrooms, onions and spices and stir until onions are translucent and mushrooms are cooked through.

This is a very tasty simple side dish, that works great on top of hamburgers, steaks, chicken - almost anything.

When I was young my brother and I would fight over who got the most of these. Yep, we fought over mushrooms.

Pictured on Page 79 Photo by Isabell Nida

Green Bean Casserole

1 lb	Organic Fresh Green Beans or Haricot Verts
2 TBSP	Organic Margarine or Olive Oil
4 oz	Organic Mushrooms – chopped
1/4 C	Organic Onion – chopped
4 oz	Organic Diary-Free Cream Cheese
1/4 C	Organic Unsweetened Non-Dairy Milk
1 TBSP	Organic Chives
1/2 tsp	Organic Garlic Powder
	Fresh Ground Salt and Pepper to taste

Preheat oven to 350 degrees. Steam your beans or verts to blanche before preparing dish.

On stovetop in skillet melt margarine or oil on medium heat. Add onions and mushrooms and cook until onions are translucent and mushrooms are soft. Set aside.

In medium mixing bowl, thoroughly mix together remaining ingredients.

In lightly greased small to medium casserole dish, layer beans, then mushroom and onion mixture and pour cream cheese mixture over top. Place in preheated oven and bake for 30 minutes.

Creamy Salsa Rice

2 C	Organic Chicken or Veggie Broth
1 C	Organic Dry Rice
1/2 TBSP	Organic Margarine
2 TBSP	Organic Dairy-Free Cream Cheese
1	Organic Tomato - minced
1 TBSP	Organic Onion - minced
1 1/2 tsp	Organic Jalapeno Pepper - minced
1 tsp	Organic Lime Juice
1 tsp	Organic Cilantro
	Fresh Ground Salt and Pepper to taste

In saucepan add rice, broth and margarine. Bring ingredients to a boil. Add in cream cheese, spices and vegetables. Lower heat to low and simmer for 15 – 20 minutes (or per package directions) until rice is soft.

Fluff with fork before serving. Serve warm.

Chicken Fried Rice

2 C	Organic Chicken Broth
1 C	Organic Dry Rice - of choice
1 TBSP	Organic Margarine
2 TBSP	Organic Olive Oil
1	Organic Egg
1/4 C	Organic Onions - chopped
1/4 C	Organic Carrots - chopped
1/4 C	Organic Petite Peas
1/4 C	Organic Mushrooms - chopped
1/4 C	Organic Zucchini - chopped
1/4 tsp	Organic Ground Ginger
1/4 tsp	Organic Ground Turmeric
1/2 tsp	Organic Ground Parsley
1/4 tsp	Organic Ground Cayenne Pepper
1/4 C	Organic Coconut Aminos
2 TBSP	Organic Margarine
1/2 lb	Organic Chicken - precooked
	Fresh Ground Salt and Pepper to taste **

In saucepan add rice, broth and margarine. Bring ingredients to a boil then lower heat to low and simmer for 15 – 20 minutes (or per package directions) until rice is soft.

Chicken Fried Rice - Continued

In large deep skillet, heat olive oil on medium heat. Add all vegetables and sauté in oil until soft – adding more oil if needed. Whisk eggs and add to pan with vegetables to fry in oil. When rice is cooked, add to pan with spices, margarine and coconut aminos, stirring to combine. Fry in pan for approximately 5 to 10 minutes, continuously stirring. Add more amino's or spices to taste.

**You can add cooked shrimp instead of chicken to change this side into Shrimp Fried Rice. I prefer to substitute a grinder of sea salt with jalapeno pepper instead of using traditional salt and pepper in this dish. It cuts the sweetness of the coconut aminos and adds a fantastic spicy flavor to this dish.

Be creative. You really can't go wrong here!

Thanksgiving Day Stuffing

1/2 loaf	Sourdough Bread – Page 125
1/2 C	Organic Rice - precooked
1/2 - 1 C	Organic Chicken or Veggie Broth
3 stalks	Organic Celery – chopped
4 oz	Organic Mushrooms - diced
1 medium	Organic Onion - minced
1/3 C	Organic Margarine - melted
2 TBSP	Organic Sage – fresh or ground
1 TBSP	Organic Parsley – fresh or ground
2 tsp	Organic Thyme – fresh or ground
	Fresh Ground Salt and Pepper to taste

Preheat oven to 350 degrees.

Pull apart sourdough bread into small shreds or cut into small pieces. Place on baking sheet and toast in your oven until they begin to brown. This may take more than one baking sheet.

Put toasted bread and precooked rice in a deep casserole dish, with a lid.

On stovetop, melt the butter on medium heat and add in mushrooms, onions and celery. Cook for five minutes. Long enough for vegetables to start to wilt.

Thanksgiving Day Stuffing - Continued

Add the cooked vegetables to casserole dish and add in spices. Use either a rubber spatula or your hands to combine, adding broth as you combine until the bread is saturated, but not wet.

Place in preheated oven for 40-45 minutes. Checking often, if top starts to burn, place the lid on casserole dish to keep from burning. Leave lid off long enough to brown the top.

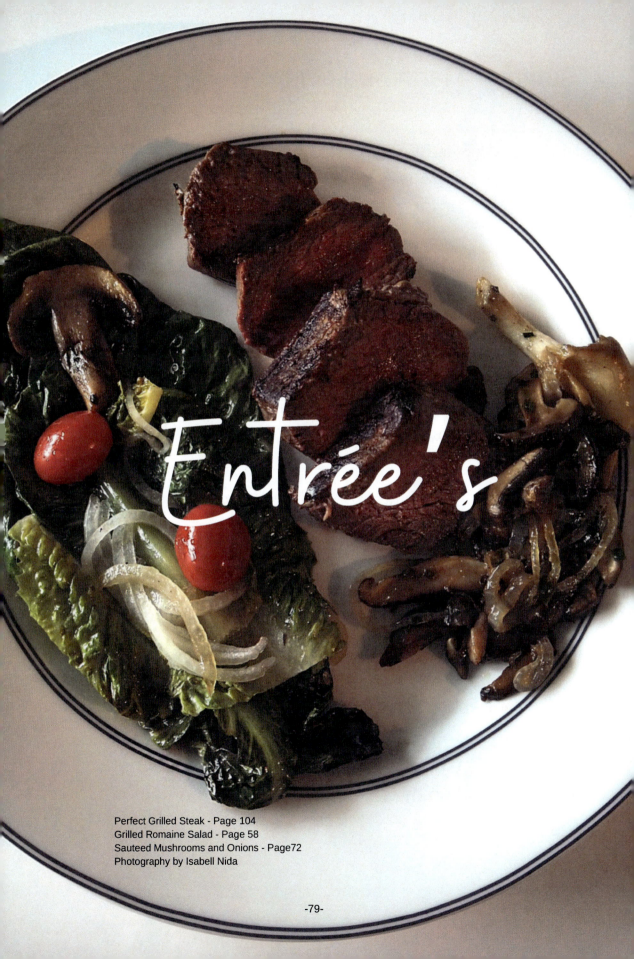

Entrée's

Perfect Grilled Steak - Page 104
Grilled Romaine Salad - Page 58
Sauteed Mushrooms and Onions - Page 72
Photography by Isabell Nida

Summer Marinated Chicken

4 -6	Organic Chicken Breasts
3 cloves	Organic Fresh Garlic - pressed
2	Organic Fresh Limes - squeezed
3 TBSP	Organic Spicy Brown Mustard
1/4 C	Coconut White Balsamic Vinegar
1/4 C	Organic Avocado or Olive Oil
1/4 C	Organic Fresh Parsley - chopped
	Fresh Ground Salt & Pepper to Taste

In a large bowl with a lid, combine all ingredients except chicken with whisk, until thoroughly mixed.

Place chicken breasts in bowl. If the marinade doesn't cover the entire chicken breast, add purified water until they are fully submerged. Place lid on bowl and put in refrigerator for 12-24 hours.

Grill until internal temperature of chicken is 170 degrees.

This is a fresh and tropical tasting marinade. Every time I make this everyone asks me for the recipe, and for whatever reason, I've never given it out – until now. Do your best to find the coconut vinegar, it the secret ingredient.

Mediterranean Chicken

4	Organic Chicken Breasts
2 TBSP	Organic Olive Oil
3 cloves	Organic Garlic - minced
1 TBSP	Mediterranean Spice - Page 45
1 TBSP	Organic Lemon Juice
1 TBSP	Lemon White Balsamic Vinegar
1/2 C	Chopped Artichoke Hearts

Place breasts in small bag and tenderize with meat tenderizer, until flattened, but still firm. Pat each breast with a paper towel to remove surface moisture. Heat oil at medium heat on stove top in a large deep skillet with a lid. Add breasts to the skillet and brown each side – About 3 minutes each. Set chicken aside.

Add garlic to pan leaving any residue from chicken to infuse with garlic. Add additional oil if needed. Add spices, lemon juice, vinegar and artichoke hearts, stirring often until it simmers. Return browned chicken breasts to pan, replace lid. Turn heat to low and let simmer for 20 – 25 minutes, until chicken is thoroughly cooked, stirring often.

Serve with Tzatziki Sauce - Page 31.

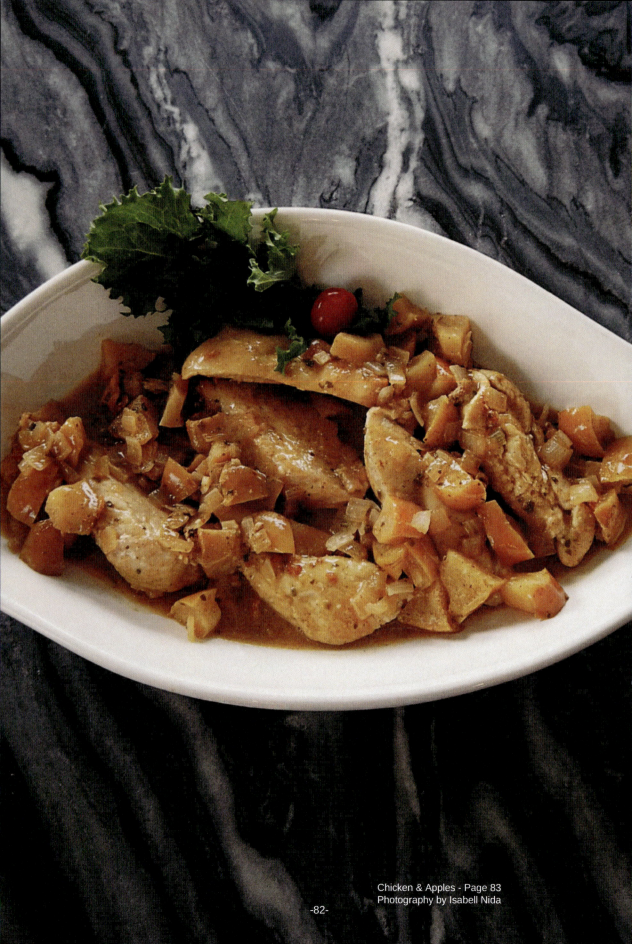

Chicken & Apples - Page 83
Photography by Isabell Nida

Chicken & Apples

Okay, at first this may not sound like a great combination, but trust me – it is!

4	Organic Boneless Chicken Breasts
2 TBSP	Organic Olive Oil
1 clove	Organic Garlic
1	Organic Onion – chopped Organic
2	Apples – cut into chunks Organic
1 C	Chicken Broth
1/4 C	Honey Mustard Sauce – Page 34
1 tsp	Organic Dried Chives
1/2 tsp	Organic Dried Parsley
1 TBSP	Organic Margarine or Coconut Oil
1 TBSP	Organic Arrowroot Flour

Preheat oven to 350 degrees.

In large enamel saucepan, heat olive oil and lightly brown both sides of each chicken breast, about 3 minutes each side. Make sure to pat each breast with a towel before adding to the pan so the oil won't splatter. Once browned, set aside.

Pictured on Page 82 - Photography by Isabell Nida

Chicken & Apples continued

Add the garlic and onions to the oil in the pan and cook until onions are translucent. Toss in the apples.

Mix the broth, honey mustard sauce and herbs in a small mixing bowl and add to pan and bring to a boil.

Place chicken breasts in pan and place in preheated oven for 20-25 minutes until breasts are thoroughly cooked through at 170 degrees interior temperature. When done, place breasts on a serving dish with the apples and onions and keep warm, reserving the liquid in the pan.

Add margarine/oil and arrowroot flour to pan with broth mixture and bring to a boil on the stove top, whisking the constantly as sauce thickens (add small amounts of additional arrowroot if needed). Once it reaches a gravy like consistency, pour over the chicken and apples and serve warm.

Goes well over rice or cauliflower rice or with your favorite vegetable.

Creamy Chicken with Artichokes

4	Organic Boneless Chicken Breasts
1/3 C	Organic Arrowroot Flour
1/4 C	Organic Margarine or Avocado Oil
1 1/2 C	Organic Dairy-Free Cream
1 C	Organic Chicken Broth
2 C	Organic Jarred Artichoke Heart
1 TBSP	Organic Lemon Juice
1 tsp	Organic Garlic Powder
1 TBSP	Organic Parsley
	Fresh Ground Salt and Pepper to taste

Place chicken in bag and tenderize with meat tenderizer. Flattening the breasts slightly, but maintaining firmness. Sprinkle each with arrowroot flour.

In large skillet, heat oil or margarine on medium heat. Place chicken in skillet and brown each side about 3 minutes each piece. Remove from pan and set aside.

In same skillet add broth and bring to a simmer. Reduce heat and simmer for 5 minutes, reducing by half. Add dairy-free cream and heat until sauce thickens. Return breasts to pan and add artichokes and salt and pepper. Place lid on pan and simmer lightly for about 10 minutes. When chicken is thoroughly cooked to 170 degrees internally, serve immediately.

Sauced Salmon

4	Wild Caught Salmon Filets*
1/2 C	Organic Mayonnaise – Page 30
1/4 C	Organic Spicy Brown or Dijon Mustard
1 TBSP	Lemon Infused White Balsamic Vinegar
1/4 tsp	Organic Garlic Powder
1 tsp	Organic Ground Parsley
	Fresh Ground Salt and Pepper to taste

Preheat oven to 350 degrees.

Place salmon (skin side down in a large baking dish, making sure they don't overlap.

In small mixing bowl, combine mayonnaise, mustard, vinegar and spices together. Pour over salmon and bake for 15 - 25 minutes (based on the thickness of the salmon filets). Serve with rice and veggies.

*You can also use this sauce with chicken breasts or cod fillets. Timing varies depending on thickness and choice of meat. This meal is super-fast and easy to make, and your family will think you're a gourmet chef. Double the sauce recipe if you want extra to pour over rice.

Seared Ahi Tuna with Sauce

8 oz	Wild Caught Ahi Tuna - block
1	Organic Jalapeno
1 bunch	Organic Fresh Cilantro
4 cloves	Organic Garlic
1/4 C	Organic Lime Juice
1/3 C	Organic Coconut Aminos
1/4 C	Organic Olive Oil
1 TBSP	Organic Ground Ginger
	Fresh Ground Salt and Pepper to taste

Mince cilantro, jalapeno and garlic and place in medium mixing bowl. Add lime juice, aminos and spices. Stir to combine well. Place in skillet and cook on medium heat for 2-3 minutes, just long enough to heat thoroughly. Set aside.

Place Ahi Tuna coated with olive oil and salt and pepper on grill mat. Preheat grill at 500-degrees. Sear each side of tuna block for about a minute to a minute and a half, ensuring that the center stays pink. Remove from grill.

Slice Tuna in 1" slices and arrange on a platter. Drizzle prepared sauce over top the tuna. Place reserve sauce in a small bowl for those who may want more. Serve immediately.

Tuna Casserole

1 lb	Fresh Wild Caught Ahi Tuna Steaks
8 oz	Organic Mushrooms - sliced
1	Organic Small Sweet Onion - chopped
3 stalks	Organic Celery - chopped
2 TBSP	Organic Fresh Parsley - chopped
1 C	Organic Peas – fresh or frozen Organic
2 TBSP	Avocado Oil
1 tsp	Organic Dried Thyme
1 1/2 tsp	Sea Salt
1/2 tsp	Organic Ground Pepper
1/3 C	Organic Unsweetened Non-Dairy Yogurt
3/4 C	Mayonnaise – Page 30
1/2 tsp	Organic Garlic Powder
1 TBSP	Organic Lemon juice
1/2 lb	Almond Flour Pasta or Zucchini Noodles

Preheat oven to 350 degrees.

Cut tuna steaks into 1" cubes. Add 1 tablespoon of oil to sauté pan, heat and add in tuna. Stir and flip constantly until cooked but still pink inside. Set aside.

Add 1 tablespoon of oil to pan and add mushrooms, onion, peas and celery until cooked, onions should appear translucent. Add spices to pan, combine and remove from heat.

Tuna Casserole - Continued

In a bowl combine the yogurt, mayonnaise, garlic powder, lemon juice and spices.

Cook zucchini noodles or almond flour pasta and place in the bottom of a 9" x 9" casserole dish. Place sautéed tuna on top, then add in vegetable mixture.

Pour sauce combination over top, mixing slightly inside of casserole dish. Cover dish with foil. Bake for 30 minutes.

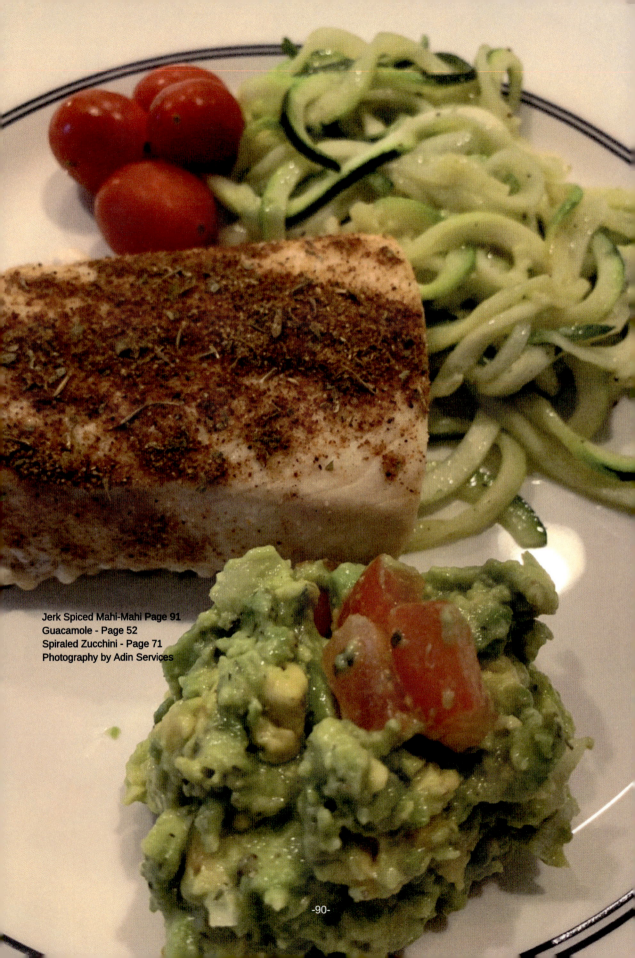

Jerk Spiced Mahi-Mahi Page 91
Guacamole - Page 52
Spiraled Zucchini - Page 71
Photography by Adin Services

Jerk Spiced Mahi-Mahi with Mango Sauce

4	Wild Caught Mahi-Mahi Filets
1 TBSP	Organic Avocado Oil
2 TBSP	Jerk Spice – Page 44
	Mango Sauce – Page 35

Preheat oven at 350 degrees.

Pat fish filets to dry and coat with jerk spice. Place in baking dish that has been brushed thoroughly with oil.

Bake at 350-degrees for 20-25 minutes. The fish will flake when cooked and will not appear pink inside.

Drizzle Mango sauce over top fish and serve.

This is one of my favorites, with or without the sauce (pictured without).

Pictured on Page 90 - Photography by Adin Services

Island Pineapple Shrimp

1 1/2 lb	Wild Caught Shrimp – shells removed
2 TBSP	Organic Avocado Oil
1/2	Organic Orange Bell Pepper
1/2	Organic Sweet Onion
1/8	Organic Pineapple – chopped
1/2 C	Organic Cherry Tomatoes
1 TBSP	Organic Parsley – fresh or ground
	Fresh Ground Salt & Pepper to taste

Pineapple Sauce – Page 36

Heat oil on stove top at medium heat. Add peppers and onions, cooking until fragrant and onions become translucent. Add in shrimp, pineapple, tomatoes and spices. Stir often, until shrimp is cooked thoroughly.

Place on plate and drizzle with pineapple sauce. Serve immediately.

This is a meal that is very tropical and refreshing. One of my summer favorites.

Crab Cakes

1 lb	Wild Caught Blue Fin Crab Meat - flaked
1	Organic Egg
1 TBSP	Organic Coconut Flour
1 TBSP	Organic Arrowroot Flour
1/4 tsp	Organic Ground Mustard
1/2 tsp	Organic Parsley Flakes
1 tsp	Old Bay Seasoning
1 TBSP	White Lemon Balsamic Vinegar
1 -2 TBSP	Organic Olive Oil, or Margarine

Ensure crab meat is free of shell fragments and place in large mixing bowl. In small bowl beat egg then add to crab. Mix well, using your hands or a rubber spatula. Add in flours, herbs and vinegar and place plastic wrap on top of bowl. Put in refrigerator for at least an hour (or overnight).

When ready to cook, divide crab mixture into 4 even cakes using your hands to mold them. Pan sear in oil of choice, ensuring both sides are browned and heated through.

Serve with tartar sauce – Page 39, or cocktail sauce – Page 40.

These are ridiculously delicious! My husband requests this dish often.

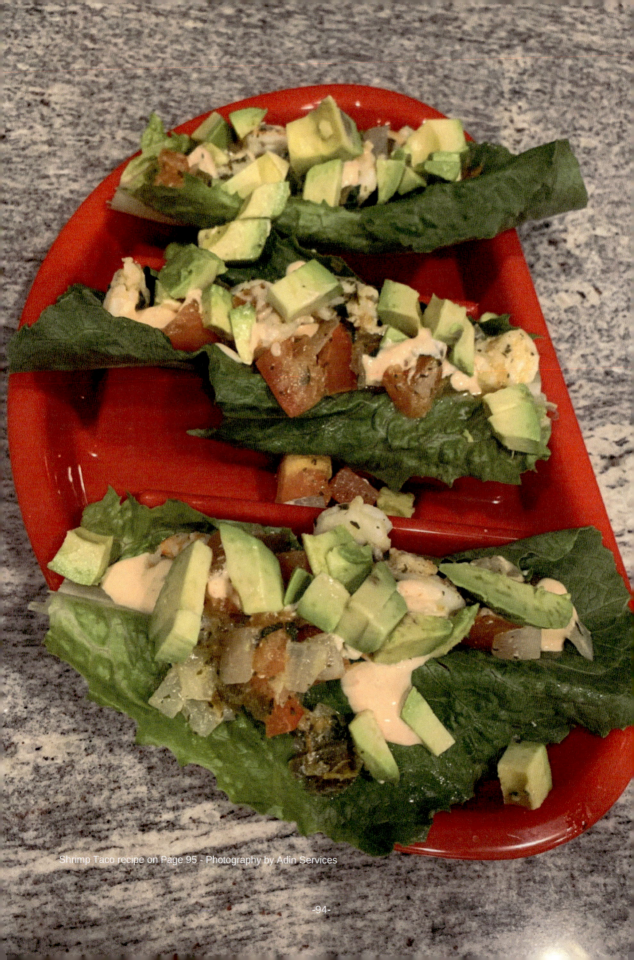

Shrimp Taco recipe on Page 95 - Photography by Adin Services

Shrimp Tacos

1 1/2 lb	Fresh Wild Caught Shrimp
2 TBSP	Organic Avocado Oil
2 TBSP	Organic Lime Juice
1/4 C	Organic Onion - minced
1	Organic Jalapeno Pepper - chopped
1	Organic Tomato - chopped
1 TBSP	Organic Cilantro
1 TBSP	Organic Parsley
1 large	Organic Avocado - chopped
	Fresh Ground Salt and pepper to taste

Sauce:

1/4 C	Organic Mayonnaise – Page 30
1-3 TBSP	Organic Hot Sauce – no sugar added
1 TBSP	Organic Lime Juice
I head	Organic Lettuce – any type

In large skillet heat oil on medium to high heat. Add minced onions and jalapeno. When onions and pepper are heated lower heat to medium low heat and add shrimp, tomatoes and spices. Continuously stir until shrimp are thoroughly cooked, yet tomatoes remain firm. Pull off heat and add chopped avocados.

Mix sauce ingredients together in small mixing bowl. Rinse individual lettuce leaves, place shrimp mixture on top of lettuce and drizzle with sauce.

Pictured on Page 94 - Photography by Adin Services

Individual Turkey Meatloaves

Loaves:

1 lb	Organic Ground Turkey
8 oz	Organic White Mushrooms - sliced
8 oz	Organic Bella Mushrooms - sliced
1/2	Organic Red Bell Pepper
1	Organic Onion - small
1/3 C	Organic Almond Flour
1	Organic Egg - beaten
1/4 C	Organic Fresh Parsley - chopped
	Fresh ground Salt and Pepper to taste

Mustard Vinaigrette:

1/2 C	Organic Spicy Brown Mustard
3 TBSP	Organic Apple Cider Vinegar
1 TBSP	Organic Dried Chives
1/4 tsp	Organic Garlic Powder
	Fresh Ground Salt and Pepper to taste

Preheat oven to 350 degrees. Lightly grease large casserole dish.

Chop mushrooms, pepper, onion, and parsley and place in large mixing bowl. Add almond flour, turkey, egg and salt and pepper to taste. Mix well with spatula. I don't recommend using your hands, as ground turkey can be very sticky.

Individual Turkey Meatloaves - continued

Use a spatula to cut mixture into quarters and sculpt into 4 mounds in lightly greased casserole dish.

Mix all vinaigrette ingredients together with whisk. Pour over the meatloaves in prepared dish. Bake in preheated oven at 350 degrees for 30 – 35 minutes.

B-B-Q Meatloaf

1 lb	Organic Ground Beef
1	Large Organic Egg
1/4 C	B-B-Q Sauce - Page 38
2 TBSP	Organic Onion - chopped
1 tsp	Organic Dried Parsley
1 tsp	Organic Dried Oregano
2 TBSP	Organic Dijon Mustard
1/4 tsp	Organic Ground Cumin
1/4 C	B-B-Q Sauce - Page 38

Preheat oven to 350 degrees.

In a large mixing bowl combine first eight ingredients either with a rubber spatula or your hands. Place in a small 6 x 8 baking dish, or mold into an oval shape in a larger dish.

Spread last half of B-B-Q sauce and over top of meatloaf.

Bake at 350 degrees for 30 – 35 minutes, until cooked thoroughly.

Baked Ziti

1 pkg	Organic Almond Flour Noodles
16 oz	Organic Pasta Sauce
1/2 lb	Organic Ground Beef - optional
8 oz	Organic Mushrooms
1	Organic Onion - small
1/2	Organic Red Bell Pepper
3 TBSP	Organic Olive Oil
8 oz	Organic Dairy-Free Cream Cheese
1/2 C	Organic Mayonnaise or Dairy-Free Yogurt
1 TBSP	Organic Dried Chives
1/2 TBSP	Organic Dried Oregano
	Fresh Ground Salt & Pepper to taste
1 C	Organic Tomatoes - diced
1/2 C	Organic Dairy-Free Shredded Cheese

Preheat oven to 350 degrees. Use olive oil to coat sides and bottom of deep casserole dish.

Cook pasta according to package directions.

In a skillet, cook the mushrooms, peppers and onions and ground beef (or leave out for vegetarian option) in olive oil until browned and beef is thoroughly cooked.

Baked Ziti - continued

In a mixing bowl combine the cream cheese, half of the shredded cheese and mayonnaise or yogurt with the dried herbs, set aside.

Layer the chopped tomatoes on the bottom of the prepared casserole dish. Put half of the cooked pasta on top, then add half of the cooked vegetables and beef mixture, top with the cheese mixture. Add the second half of the pasta on top of the cheese, then the next half of the vegetables and pour the pasta sauce over entire pan and top with the last half of the shredded cheese - optional.

Cook for 35 – 45 Minutes at 350 degrees. Timing will depend on how deep your dish is.

I've made this for several family functions and everyone wants the recipe, but I don't give it out because they don't know it's gluten and dairy free!

Stewed Flat Iron Steaks

4	Grass Fed Organic Flat Iron Steaks
2 TBSP	Organic Olive Oil
1	Organic Onion - sliced
3 cloves	Organic Garlic - minced
2 1/2 C	Organic Tomatoes – diced
2 tsp	Organic Ground Cumin
2 C	Organic Beef Broth/Stock
	Fresh Ground Salt and Pepper to taste

Preheat oven to 350 degrees.

In large enamel skillet with lid, heat olive oil on medium high heat. Pat steaks with paper towel to remove excess exterior moisture, put in hot skillet and brown both sides, at least 2 minutes per steak. Set aside – keep warm.

In same skillet, add onions and garlic and cook in fats until onion is translucent and garlic is fragrant. Add tomatoes, spices and broth and bring to a boil.

Add steaks to skillet, making sure to allow juice from pan to flow around them, and place in the oven for 2 hours with the lid on.

Stewed Flat Iron Steaks - continued

Remove skillet from oven and place steaks in large shallow bowl or on a cutting board and use forks to shred the meat. Place shredded meat back into pan and stir to combine with sauce and vegetables. Place in dish and serve warm.

This is a simple recipe, but it has a big impact. The steak melts in your mouth and the flavors work beautifully together.

I typically serve this over mashed potatoes or rice with a vegetable side.

Meatballs

1 lb	Organic Ground Beef or Turkey
2 slices	Sourdough Bread – Page 125 – toasted
1	Organic Onion - minced
1	Organic Egg
1 tsp	Organic Dried Oregano
1 tsp	Organic Dried Basil
1/2 tsp	Organic Dried Thyme
1/4 tsp	Organic Garlic Powder
1/4 tsp	Organic Ground Mustard Powder
	Fresh Ground Salt and Pepper to taste

Preheat oven to 350 degrees.

Combine all ingredients in large mixing bowl. Use rubber spatula or your hands to combine thoroughly.

Using 1" scooper, scoop into balls and place on baking sheet or in a large casserole dish, making sure they don't touch.

Cook in oven at 350 degrees for 20-25 minutes, until cooked through.

Serve as is, or over gluten free pasta or rice. I like to make wilted spinach and put my meatballs on top and drizzle with olive oil and pine nuts. Be creative!

Perfectly Grilled Steak

4 6-8 oz   Organic Grass Fed Steaks - your choice
3 TBSP   Organic Margarine
              Freshly Ground Salt and Pepper to taste

If you've got high quality organic beef for this recipe, you're golden.

Melt the margarine. Place steaks on grill mat and drizzle the melted margarine overtop them. Sprinkle with salt and pepper.

Grill for 4 minutes each side for 1" thick steaks. Add another minute per side for each additional ¼".

Let sit for 2 minutes before serving. Should be cooked to a perfect medium rare steak.

Pair this with my Grilled Romaine Salad, Page 58, it's delicious!

Sometimes the simplest recipes are the best!

Pictured on Page 79 - Photography by Isabell Nida

SOUP

Creamy Shrimp Chowder - Recipe on Page 107
Fluffy Sandwich Bread - Recipe on Page 128
Photography by Adin Services

Chicken Noodle Soup

3 stalks	Organic Celery
3	Organic Carrots
2 cloves	Organic Garlic
1	Organic Onion
1 1/2 lb	Organic Chicken - pre-cooked Organic
48 oz	Chicken Broth/Stock
3-4 TBSP	Organic Olive Oil
1 C	Organic Gluten-Free Pasta or Rice
1/4 C	Organic Fresh Parsley
	Fresh Ground Salt and Pepper to taste

In large soup pot add oil, onion, garlic, celery and carrots. Sauté on high until onions are translucent and garlic is aromatic.

Add broth or stock and leave on high heat until boiling. Once boiling add cooked chopped or shredded chicken. If you're in a huge hurry canned organic chicken breast will do the trick!

Bring back to boiling, then add noodles, salt pepper and parsley and cook for 10 - 20 minutes on medium heat until noodles are cooked.

Serve warm with a slice of Sourdough bread, Page 125.

Creamy Shrimp Chowder

1 lb	Wild Caught Shrimp – cooked & chopped
2 TBSP	Organic Olive Oil
1/2 C	Organic Celery - chopped
1/2 C	Organic Mushrooms - sliced
1/3 C	Organic Onion - diced
1 C	Organic Russet Potatoes - cubed
1 1/2 C	Organic Vegetable Broth
1 1/2 C	Organic Unsweetened Non-Dairy Milk
6 oz	Organic Non-Dairy Cream Cheese
1 TBSP	Organic Lemon Juice
1 1/2 tsp	Organic Creole Seasoning
1 TBSP	Organic Parsley
1	Bay Leaf
	Fresh Ground Salt and Pepper to taste

In a large pot sauté celery, onions and mushrooms in olive oil. Cook until onions are translucent stirring frequently, add broth, milk and cream cheese to pot. Stir until smooth and thoroughly combined.

Add potatoes, shrimp, lemon juice, bay leaf and spices. Place on low heat and simmer for 20-30 minutes at a low boil, stirring occasionally.

Remove bay leaf and serve warm.

Pictured on Page 105 - Photography by Adin Services

Creamy Tomato Dill Soup

2	Organic Vidalia Onions
3 cloves	Organic Garlic
2 TBSP	Organic Olive Oil
2 TBSP	Organic Lemon Juice
2 C	Organic Chicken or Vegetable Broth
3-14 oz	Organic Tomato Sauce - canned
1-14 oz	Organic Diced Tomato - canned
3/4 C	Organic Dairy-Free Heavy Cream
1 TBSP	Organic Arrowroot Flour
1 TBSP	Organic Dried Dill Weed
	Fresh Ground Salt and Pepper to taste

Chop onions and place in food processor, until onions are finely chopped. Place in warm soup pot with olive oil and simmer on medium heat. Chop garlic and add once onions become fragrant. Cook for two minutes, do not brown. Add stock or broth, canned tomatoes and lemon juice all at once and bring to a boil. Turn down heat to keep at a low boil, leave simmer for 30 minutes.

In measuring cup combine diary-free cream and arrowroot flour. Whisk until smooth, then add dill weed, salt & pepper. Add cream mixture to pot, ensure no lumps from flour remains. Simmer for 10 minutes, on low, stirring often.
Serve warm.

Italian Beef Soup

1 lb	Organic Grass Fed Ground Beef
1 TBSP	Organic Olive Oil
1/2 C	Organic Onion
2 Cloves	Organic Garlic
2	Organic Tomatoes - chopped
1/4 tsp	Organic Dried Parsley
1/4 tsp	Organic Dried Oregano
1/4 tsp	Organic Dried Basil
4 C	Organic Beef Broth or Stock
8 oz	Organic Rice

Chop onions and garlic into small pieces. Heat oil on stovetop at medium heat. Add onion and garlic and cook until onions are translucent and the garlic is aromatic. Add beef and stir often to break down large clumps. You want the beef to be a crumble texture. Once beef is cooked thoroughly, pour off excess oil and fats.

Chop tomatoes into small pieces and add to beef mixture with herbs and broth. Bring to a boil on medium-high heat.

Stir in the pasta or rice and reduce heat slightly, cook for 10 – 20 minutes, according to package directions, until pasta or rice is done.

Serve with a slice of Sourdough bread, Page 125.

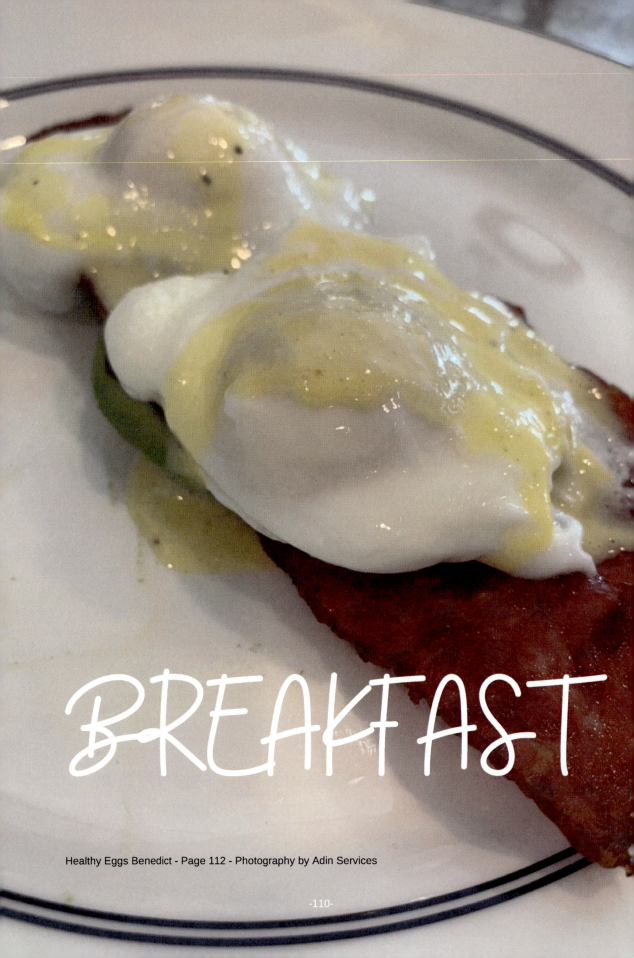

BREAKFAST

Healthy Eggs Benedict - Page 112 - Photography by Adin Services

Pancake Mix – Grain Free

3/4 C   Organic Almond Flour
1/2 C   Organic Arrowroot Flour
1/4 C   Organic Coconut Palm Sugar
2 TBSP   Organic Coconut Flour
1 tsp   Cream of Tartar
1/2 tsp   Baking Soda
1/2 tsp   Sea Salt

Mix all ingredients and store in an air-tight container until ready to make.

For 2 - six-inch pancakes use: 1/4 C Pancake Mix, 1 Organic Egg, 1 TBSP, Organic Unsweetened Non-Diary Milk, 1/2 TBSP, Organic Avocado Oil

For 6 - six-inch pancakes use: 1 1/2 C Pancake Mix, 3 Organic Eggs, 3 TBSP Organic Unsweetened Non-Dairy Milk, 2 TBSP Organic Avocado Oil

For 10 - six-inch pancakes use: 2 1/4 C Pancake Mix, 5 Organic Eggs, 1/3 C Organic Unsweetened Non-Dairy Milk, 3 TBSP Organic Olive Oil

Combine all ingredients and place batter on hot skillet with avocado oil and fry both sides to ensure thoroughly cooked. Top with margarine, maple syrup, berries or your choice of topping.

Healthy Eggs Benedict

Hollandaise Sauce
1/2 C	Organic Margarine
1 TBSP	Organic Lemon Juice
3	Organic Egg Yolks
	Fresh Ground Salt and Pepper to taste
6 slices	Organic Turkey Bacon
6	Organic Eggs
2	Ripe Organic Avocados

In a small saucepan melt margarine on low heat. Keep on heat after it melts until it starts to bubble, but not brown.

In your blender add egg yolks, lemon juice, salt and pepper and process to combine. While the egg mixture is running, add the hot margarine in a slow stream from top. When margarine is fully incorporated, turn off the blender and set aside, sealing top with lid.

Turkey Bacon:

In a roasting pan lay the strips of turkey bacon on the rack and bake at 400 degrees until desired crispness 15-25 minutes.

Pictured on Page 110 - Photography by Adin Services

Healthy Eggs Benedict - continued

Avocado:
Slice the avocados.

Poached Eggs:

In a large but shallow pan fill 2/3 full with water. Set on stovetop at medium to high heat until water boils. Drop eggs into boiling water one at a time. You can add vinegar to the water to keep the eggs together while cooking – but it does add a vinegar flavor to the dish. I just toss them in the water – bombs away style, as I'm not so picky as to how round they turn out. You can also use a poaching pan if you're particular. Cook the eggs until the whites are thoroughly cooked and the yolk is still liquid. Remove eggs from water with slotted spoon, ensure you don't overcook them.

On your plate layer the sliced avocado, the turkey bacon, then place the poached egg on top of bacon and pour hollandaise sauce on top.

This is a great dish for special occasions, we make this for birthdays, and almost every holiday breakfast and of course, on days where it just feels appropriate.

French Toast

1 Loaf	Sourdough Bread – Page 125
1/2 C	Organic Unsweetened Non-Dairy Milk
1	Organic Egg
1 tsp	Organic Ground Cinnamon
	Organic Margarine

Slice bread in desired thickness.

In a shallow bowl whisk egg, milk and cinnamon.

Soak bread slices in egg mixture for about sixty seconds, ensuring both sides are coated.

Place on hot greased griddle and fry both sides, about 2 minutes per side, but you can go longer or less depending on how brown you want your French Toast to be.

Pat with a small amount of margarine and top with your favorite topping.

Topping suggestions:

Organic maple syrup – vanilla bean infused is a great option for this. Fruit spread – sweetened only with fruit, or fresh organic berries.

Hash Browns

2	Organic Russet Potatoes – pre-baked
2 TBSP	Organic Onion
1/4	Organic Bell Pepper - optional
1 TBSP	Organic Olive Oil
2 TBSP	Organic Margarine
1/2 tsp	Organic Garlic Powder
	Fresh Ground Salt and Pepper to taste

Grate your pre-baked potatoes onto large cutting board on largest grate setting. Grate onion on top of potatoes on smallest grate setting. Dice peppers.

Heat olive oil on cast iron griddle or large skillet on high. Add chopped and grated vegetables to griddle, add spices and margarine. With a metal spatula, flip and stir on griddle until golden brown.

Serve immediately.

I like to top the hash browns with fried eggs.

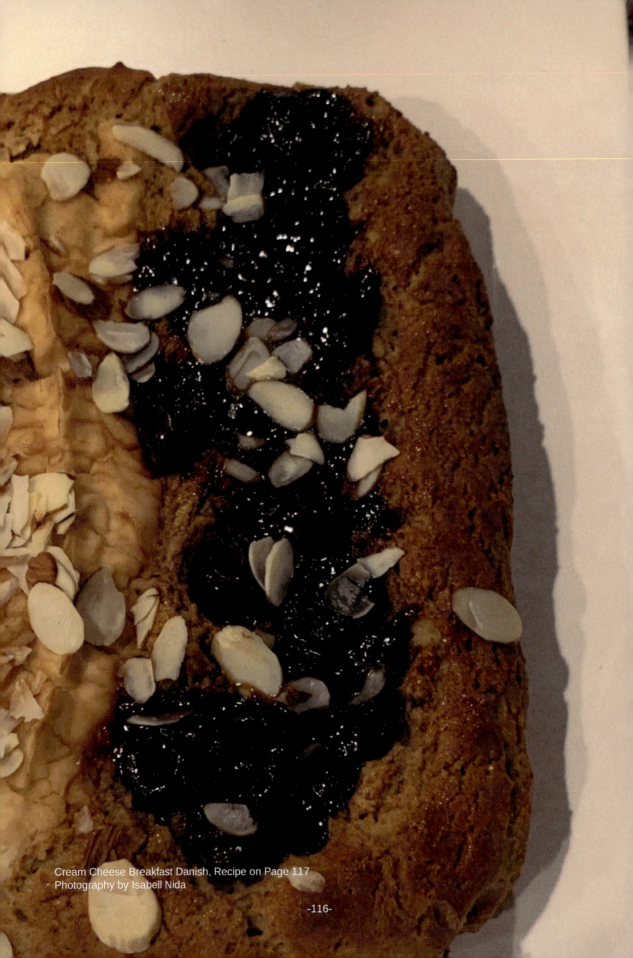

Cream Cheese Breakfast Danish, Recipe on Page 117
Photography by Isabell Nida

Cream Cheese Breakfast Danish

1/4 C	Hot Water
1/4 C	Organic Unsweetened Dairy-Free Milk
2 1/4 tsp	Organic Dry Yeast
1/2 C	Organic Sorghum Flour
1/4 C	Organic Tapioca Flour
1/4 C	Organic Brown Rice Flour
1/4 C	Organic White Rice Flour
1/3 C	Organic Coconut Palm Sugar
1/2 tsp	Xanthan Gum
1/4 tsp	Sea Salt
1	Organic Egg
2 TBSP	Organic Coconut Oil - melted
1 TBSP	Organic Coconut Palm Sugar
1/3 C	Organic Dairy-Free Cream Cheese
1 TBSP	Organic Raw Honey
1 C	Frozen Organic Cherries
1 TBSP	Organic Arrowroot Flour
2 TBSP	Organic Coconut Palm Sugar
1 TBSP	Raw Slivered Almonds

Preheat oven to 350 degrees.

Pictured on Page 116 - Photography by Isabell Nida

Cream Cheese Breakfast Danish - continued

In measuring cup add hot water and milk – don't stir, sprinkle dry yeast on top and let it proof – set aside.

Mix all dry ingredients in standing mixture. Add melted oil, egg and proofed yeast to mixer on low until combined. Turn up to high for 5 minutes, scraping sides of bowl often.

Line a 9" x 4" loaf pan or baking dish with parchment paper. Add dough and sprinkle top with coconut palm sugar. Place plastic wrap on top and set aside to rise for 45 minutes – 1 hour.

While rising, combine cream cheese and honey in a small bowl. Set aside.

On the stove top, combine the frozen cherries, arrowroot flour and coconut palm sugar in a small skillet. Set heat on medium low and stir constantly until cherries are soft and the juice starts to thicken. Set aside.

Once the dough has risen, use a sharp knife to cut the top down the sides in two lines. Place cream cheese in one slit, and the cherries in the other slit. Sprinkle top with slivered almonds.

Cream Cheese Breakfast Danish - Continued

Bake at 350 degrees for 35-45 minutes.

To make an Apple Cream Cheese Danish, switch the frozen cherries with a chopped apple, and add a tsp of coconut oil, continue as directed.

To make a Chocolate Cream Cheese Danish, in a small sauce pan on very low heat, add ¼ C of organic no cane sugar chocolate chips and 2 tsp of organic coconut oil and a 1/4 tsp of vanilla extract until melted and pour into the second slit and cook as directed.

Be creative. This danish can be any flavor you want!

BREADS

Raisin Bread Recipe - Page 130
Photography by Isabell Nida

Gluten Free Sourdough Starter

Keep in mind you need to start this recipe at least three days (preferably five days) before you want to make sourdough bread! Plan accordingly, or else you'll be very disappointed in your results.

1 TBSP	Organic Active Dry Yeast
1 C	Organic Unsweetened Diary-Free Milk
1/2 C	Organic White Rice Flour
1/2 C	Gluten Free Flour Mix – Page 123
1 tsp	Organic Raw Honey

In a glass measuring bowl combine milk and honey. Place in microwave for 30 seconds to heat slightly. Add in active dry yeast and stir until dissolved.

In a larger glass bowl with a lid (I use Pyrex bowls) add in flours and mix thoroughly. Add warm milk to flour mixture and combine thoroughly.

Leave on your counter at room temperature for three to five days, stirring twice a day. Keep it covered. While you wait, you're fermenting the starter and this process takes time, so try to be patient. You may see the mixture bubble, usually in the beginning, I've even had it pop the lid off my container and make a mess on my counter. It could also separate in the bowl; this is all

Gluten Free Sourdough Starter - continued

normal. Leave it out on the counter at room temperature until it's ready to feed. If you feed it too early, it won't taste right.

HOW TO FEED:

FIRST FEEDING: Stir starter well before feeding. Add 3/4 cup of white rice and 3/4 cup of gluten free flour mix, as well as 3/4 cup of warm water (approximately 100 degrees). Stir to mix thoroughly and use immediately. If not thin enough, just add a tablespoon at a time of water until you get the right consistency. After your first use, store the starter in your refrigerator. Your starter can be re-fed and used for months, some people have even said they have starter that is decades old. The only way you'll need to start over is if it turns color or smells. You'll know instinctively if your starter has gone bad. After each use you need to re-feed your starter.

TO RE-FEED:

Add 1/2 cup of white rice flour and 1/2 cup of gluten free flour mix and 1/2 to 3/4 cup of warm water (approximately 100 Degrees). Leave on counter overnight. Stir and refrigerate in the morning until your next use.

Gluten Free Flour Mix

1 1/2 C	Organic Brown Rice Flour
1 C	Organic Tapioca Flour
1 C	Organic White Rice Flour
1/2 C	Organic Cassava Flour
1/2 C	Organic Sorghum Flour
1/2 C	Organic Arrowroot Flour
2 TBSP	Organic Psyllium Husk Powder
2 tsp	Organic Guar Gum

In a very large bowl, mix all ingredients until well combined. Store in an air-tight container in your pantry in climate-controlled conditions.

I usually double this recipe when I make it, as I go through this flour mix quickly, as sourdough bread is a staple in my family. I do not suggest making any substitutions, as this recipe has taken me months to perfect and creates a delicious result.

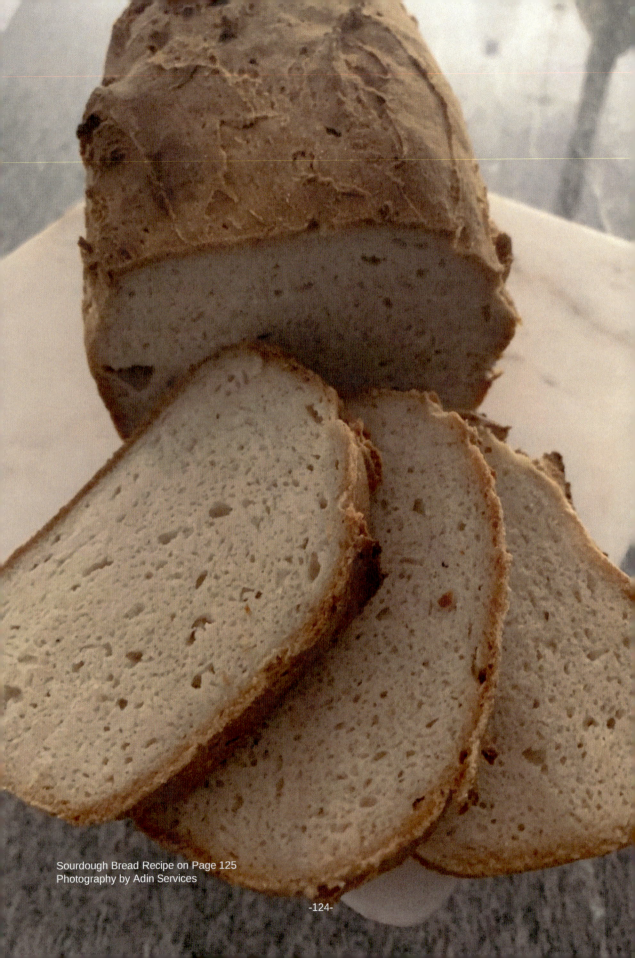

Sourdough Bread Recipe on Page 125
Photography by Adin Services

Sourdough Bread

2 1/2 C	Gluten Free Flour Mix – Page 123
1/2 C	Organic Almond Flour
2 1/4 tsp	Organic Dry Yeast
1 1/4 tsp	Baking Powder - aluminum free
1 1/2 tsp	Sea Salt
1/4 tsp	Cream of Tartar
1 C	"FED" Sourdough Starter
1 1/2 C	Organic Unsweetened Dairy-Free Milk
2 tsp	Xanthan Gum
1/2 tsp	Guar Gum
1 TBSP	Organic Raw Honey
3 TBSP	Organic Coconut Oil - melted

Preheat oven at 400 degrees.

In a glass measuring cup (2 Cups or larger) add the milk and honey. Microwave for one minute to bring to 100 degrees. Add the xanthan gum and guar gum to the milk mixture and whisk (this will be lumpy – it's okay).

Place coconut oil in microwave safe dish and melt, approximately 30 seconds.

Pictured on Page 124 - Photography by Adin Services

Sourdough Bread - continued

In standing mixer, add all dry ingredients and place on low speed. When combined add in the sourdough starter, then milk mixture and coconut oil. Leave on low until completely combined. Once combined, beat on medium/high speed for five minutes, using a rubber spatula to scrape the sides often.

While the dough is beating, get out your bread pan 9" x 4" and line with parchment paper. I usually place the pan on top of the parchment paper and cut it from the edge to the corner of the pan on all 4 corners and fold it together to create a tight liner.

When the mixing is complete, place dough into lined pan spreading evenly. I use a rubber spatula, but if you use your hands, wet them first. The dough is sticky and thick at this point.

Place a clean dry towel over bread and leave to rise for 1 to 1 ½ hours in a warm dry place.

Bake at 400 degrees for 45-50 minutes, until top is lightly brown.

Do not cut into this bread until it has cooled, otherwise it might still be tacky and you can make a mess out of it.

Sourdough Bread - continued

This sourdough has an amazing flavor and is worth the wait, as it comes out with a nice crispy brown crust with a fluffy inside. It is absolutely delicious!

Store it in a zip-lock storage bag, and since it never lasts more than a few days, I do not refrigerate it. It should stay fresh for 6-7 days stored at room temperature.

This is my absolute favorite bread!

At the first sign that it is starting to go stale, make french toast! – Page 114.

Fluffy Sandwich Bread

1 C	Organic Sorghum Flour
1/2 C	Organic Tapioca Flour
1/2 C	Organic Brown Rice Flour
1/3 C	Organic White Rice Flour
1/4 C	Organic Coconut Palm Sugar
1 tsp	Xanthan Gum
1 tsp	Sea Salt
1/2 C	Hot Purified Water
1/2 C	Organic Unsweetened Non-Dairy Milk
1 1/2 TBSP	Organic Active Dry Yeast
2	Organic Large eggs
1/3 C	Organic Coconut Oil - melted

Preheat oven to 350 degrees. Line 9" x 5" Bread loaf pan with parchment paper.

Combine hot water and milk in glass measuring cup and sprinkle the yeast on top– let sit to proof.

Add all dry ingredients into bowl of stand mixer. Combine on low speed.

Pictured on Page 105 - Photography by Adin Services

Fluffy Sandwich Bread - continued

Add eggs and coconut oil to proofed yeast mixture, then add to standing mixer with dry ingredients. Combine thoroughly on low setting, then place on high and mix for 5 minutes, scraping bowl occasionally.

Put dough directly into parchment lined loaf pan (dough will be thin, like cake batter) and wrap cellophane over top of the loaf pan, leave room for expansion. Set aside to rise for 1 to 1 ½ hours, until loaf doubles.

Bake on center rack at 350 degrees for 50-55 minutes.

This bread can be eaten immediately after it comes out of the oven. Beautifully buttery flavored, fluffy bread that no one would ever guess is gluten free.

Keeps for about a week in an airtight bag/container and does not need to be refrigerated.

Raisin Bread

1 C	Organic Sorghum Flour
1/2 C	Organic Tapioca Flour
1/2 C	Organic Brown Rice Flour
1/3 C	Organic White Rice Flour
2/3 C	Organic Coconut Palm Sugar
1 TBSP	Organic Ground Cinnamon
1 tsp	Xanthan Gum
1 tsp	Sea Salt
1/2 C	Hot Purified Water
1/2 C	Organic Unsweetened Non-Diary Milk
1 1/2 TBSP	Organic Active Dry Yeast
2	Organic Eggs
1/3 C	Organic Coconut oil - melted
3/4 C	Organic Raisins
3 TBSP	Organic Coconut Palm Sugar
1 TBSP	Organic Ground Cinnamon
1/4 tsp	Organic Ground Cardamon (optional)

Preheat oven to 350 degrees. Line 9" x 5" loaf pan with parchment paper.

Pictured on Page 120 - Photography by Isabell Nida

Raisin Bread - continued

In a small bowl add raisins and submerge in very warm water (not boiling) to let soak while preparing bread.

Combine hot water and milk in glass measuring cup, sprinkle the yeast on top – set aside to proof.

Add all dry ingredients to the bowl of standing mixer. Turn on lowest speed to combine.

Add eggs and coconut oil to the proofed yeast mixture and combine. Add liquids to dry ingredients and mix on low setting until thoroughly combined. Turn on high setting for 5 minutes scraping sides of bowl occasionally.

In small bowl, combine the coconut palm sugar, cinnamon and cardamon for sprinkling.

Drain raisins.

When dough is ready, layer into pre-lined loaf pan. Add 1/3 of dough directly to parchment lined loaf pan (dough may be thin like cake batter). Add half of the raisins, then 1/3 of the sugar/cinnamon. Add second layer of dough, the last of the raisins and 1/3 of the sugar/cinnamon.

Raisin Bread - continued

Finally add the last third of the dough and sprinkle with the last of the sugar/cinnamon. Wrap cellophane over top of pan leaving room for expansion.

Set aside to rise for 1 to 1 1/2 hours, until loaf doubles.

Bake on center rack at 350 degrees for 50-55 minutes.

The bread can be eaten immediately after it comes out of the oven. Crispy crust with a sweet and fluffy cinnamon raisin center. Absolutely delicious!

Keeps for about a week in an airtight bag/container and does not need to be refrigerated.

Flat Bread

1 1/2 C   Gluten Free Flour Mix – Page 123
1/4 C   Organic Almond Flour
3 TBSP   Nutritional Yeast
3/4 tsp   Sea Salt
1 1/2 tsp   Baking Powder - aluminum free
3 TBSP   Organic Olive Oil
3/4 C   Organic Unsweetened Non-Diary Milk

Mix all dry ingredients in medium bowl.

Measure milk and oil in measuring cup and combine. Pour wet ingredients into dry ingredients and stir until smooth.

Make four balls of dough and lay out on a pastry mat. Use the palm of your hand or a rubber spatula to flatten balls into 6-8" circles.

Heat griddle or skillet on stove top on medium heat, adding a TBSP or so of olive oil to grease pan. Fry each circle of dough until golden brown, flipping over to cook evenly.

I love serving this bread with Grilled Chicken covered in Tzatziki sauce, accompanied by a small salad.

Apple Cinnamon Muffins – Grain Free

These are so simple and flavorful and don't require a lot of effort. I love having these around for breakfast or a snack.

1 1/4 C	Organic Almond Flour
3 TBSP	Organic Coconut Flour
1/2 tsp	Baking Soda
1/4 tsp	Sea Salt
1 TBSP	Organic Ground Cinnamon
2	Organic Eggs
1/3 C	Organic Coconut Oil
1/3 C	Organic Raw Honey
1 tsp	Organic Vanilla Extract
1/2 C	Organic Apple - grated
1 C	Organic Apple - diced
1/4 C	Organic Raisins
1/4 C	Walnuts - chopped

Preheat oven to 350 degrees.

In a medium mixing bowl, combine all dry ingredients from almond flour to cinnamon together and set aside.

In a large bowl add all wet ingredients and stir to combine. Add the dry ingredients to the wet mixture and stir by hand until completely combined.

Apple Cinnamon Muffins - continued

Add in the diced and grated apples, raisins and walnuts, pour into lined cupcake tins.

Bake for 25 minutes on middle rack. Check using a toothpick that comes out clean before removing from oven. Cool on wire rack.

If you decide to make these in muffin-sized tins, add 10-15 minutes to your baking time.

Orange Cranberry Bread – Grain Free

1 C	Organic Almond Flour
1/3 C	Organic Coconut Flour
1/2 tsp	Baking Soda
1/4 tsp	Sea Salt
1 TBSP	Organic Orange Zest
3	Organic Eggs
1/3 C	Organic Raw Honey
2 TBSP	Organic Avocado Oil
1 tsp	Organic Vanilla Extract
1/4 C	Organic Orange Juice
1/2 C	Organic Dried Unsweetened Cranberries

Preheat oven to 350 degrees. Line a 9" x 4" loaf pan with parchment paper.

In large bowl combine all dry ingredients, make a well in the center.

In smaller bowl thoroughly combine all wet ingredients. Slowly beat wet ingredients into dry ingredients in large bowl. Add in chopped cranberries and let sit for 5 minutes.

Orange Cranberry Bread – continued

Put dough in lined pan and place in the middle rack of oven. Cook for 40–50 minutes, test with knife or toothpick before removing from oven, to ensure bread is done.

Place on wire rack with parchment paper and cool for 20-30 minutes before serving. Can be served warm or chilled.

Keep stored in refrigerator in air-tight container.

Switch the orange zest and juice with lemon zest and juice and switch the cranberries with blueberries and you have Lemon Blueberry Bread, which is just as delicious!

Pizza Dough

1/2 C	Hot Purified Water- about 110 degrees
2 TBSP	Organic Coconut Palm Sugar
1 TBSP	Organic Active Dry Yeast
2 1/2 tsp	Organic Apple Cider Vinegar
2	Organic Egg Whites
1/4 C	Organic Olive Oil
1 C	Organic Tapioca Flour
1/2 C	Organic Almond Flour
1/2 C	Organic Brown Rice Flour
1 1/2 tsp	Xanthan Gum
1/2 tsp	Sea Salt
1/2 tsp	Baking Powder

In measuring cup add hot water, coconut palm sugar and yeast, set aside.

In standing mixer whisk egg whites on high for approximately 3 minutes, until medium-stiff peaks form. Add the vinegar and oil to the yeast mixture, stir and add to the egg whites. Turn mixer on low for about a minute to combine ingredients, don't over mix. Over mixing is counter-productive to whisking the egg whites.

Pizza Dough - continued

In a medium bowl, add dry ingredients together and stir. Turn on mixer to low add dry ingredients to the egg mixture, not too fast, not too slow. Once combined stop mixing and set aside.

Grease a large pizza pan - 18" or two smaller 9" pans, dump dough onto pan and work with your fingers or a rubber spatula to push to the edge. Keep dough evenly distributed in pan. Place clean dishcloth over pan(s) and set aside 30 minutes to rise. At this time, preheat oven to 400 degrees.

When the dough has risen, top with sauce – Page 35, and add toppings of your choice. Place in the middle rack of your oven for 20-25 minutes to bake. Crust should be crunchy on the bottom but light and fluffy inside.

SMOOTHIES

Banana Nut Smoothing - Top - Recipe on Page 142
Cherry Smoothie - Bottom - Recipe on Page 141
Photography by Adin Services

I use frozen fruits in my smoothies, that way I do not have to add ice, and therefore they are more flavorful. It's a great way to keep from throwing away fruit that's about to over ripen. If I cut up a pineapple and I notice I don't have much time to finish it, I throw it in a freezer bag and put it in the freezer for smoothies. This works well for almost any fruit!

I also use pea protein powder in my smoothies. Most protein powders on the market are full of unwanted ingredients. The simpler it is, the more likely I will not react to it. Organic Pea Protein is easy to find and is not expensive.

Cherry Smoothie

1/2 C	Frozen Organic Sweet Cherries
1 C	Organic Unsweetened Dairy-Free Milk
2 TBSP	Organic Protein Powder
2 -3 TBSP	Organic Nut Butter (use your favorite)

Place all ingredients into a blender and mix until smooth.

Pictured on Page 140 - Photography by Adin Services

Chocolate Cherry Smoothie

It's the same as the cherry smoothie, but you add 1 ½ TBSP of organic cocoa powder. You might find this bitter if you're not used to unsweetened smoothies. You can add organic raw honey or coconut palm sugar if you want. I do not recommend sweetening smoothies, but you might prefer them that way.

Banana Nut Smoothie

1/2 C	Frozen Organic Bananas
1 C	Organic Unsweetened Dairy-Free Milk
2 TBSP	Organic Protein Powder
2 -3 TBSP	Organic Nut Butter (use your favorite)

Place all ingredients into a blender and mix until smooth.

Pictured on Page 140 - Photography by Adin Services

Pina Colada Smoothie

1/2 C	Frozen Organic Pineapple
1/2 C	Organic Coconut Milk (from a can)
1/2 C	Organic Unsweetened Dairy-Free Milk
2 TBSP	Organic Protein Powder
2 -3 TBSP	Nut Butter (use your favorite)

Place all ingredients into a blender and mix until smooth. This one is so refreshing and sometimes I add frozen mango or strawberries to it on occasion as well. YUM!

Berry Smoothie

1/2 C	Organic Frozen Mixed Berries
1 C	Organic Unsweetened Dairy-Free Milk
2 TBSP	Organic Protein Powder
2 -3 TBSP	Organic Nut Butter (use your favorite)

Place all ingredients into a blender and mix until smooth.

Chocolate Nut Butter Chia Smoothie

1 C	Organic Unsweetened Dairy-Free Milk
2 TBSP	Organic Protein Powder
2 TBSP	Organic Raw Cocoa Powder
2 -3 TBS	Organic Nut Butter (use your favorite)
2 TBSP	Organic Chia Seeds
1/2 C	Ice

Place all ingredients into a blender and mix until smooth. As with the Chocolate Cherry Smoothie, you might want to add a sweetener to this one. Ice is needed as there isn't any frozen fruit in this smoothie to make it the right temperature or consistency.

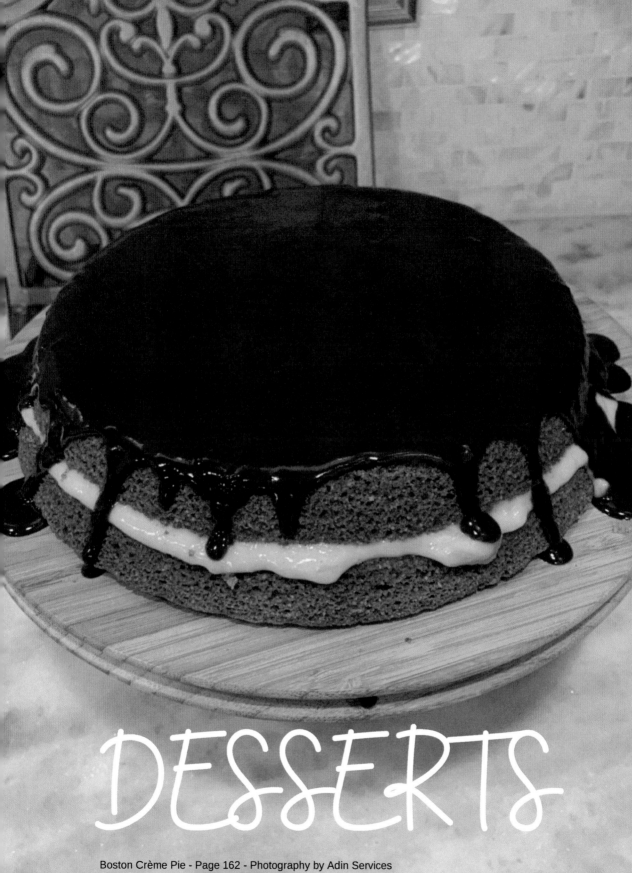

DESSERTS

Boston Crème Pie - Page 162 - Photography by Adin Services

Chocolate Silk Pie

3/4 C	Organic Coconut Palm Sugar
1/4 C	Organic Corn Starch
3 TBSP	Organic Unsweetened Cocoa Powder
1/4 tsp	Sea Salt
1 C	Organic Coconut Crème - canned
2 C	Organic Unsweetened Non-Dairy Milk
3	Organic Egg Yolks
1 tsp	Organic Vanilla Extract
2 TBSP	Organic Margarine
1 C	Organic Chocolate Chips
2 oz	100% Organic Dark Chocolate - solid

In a medium saucepan add all dry ingredients from coconut palm sugar through sea salt. Whisk in ½ cup coconut crème and ½ cup non-dairy milk until thoroughly combined. Place on medium to low heat and slowly add in the rest of the milk and crème along with the egg yolks, whisking continuously. Bring to a low boil, let boil for one minute.

Remove from heat and whisk in margarine, vanilla and solid chocolate. Whisk until the chocolates have melted and the mixture is smooth.

Chocolate Silk Pie - continued

Place in prepared Graham Cracker Pie Crust - Page 149 and place plastic wrap directly on top of the pie filling. This keeps the pie from forming a skin as a top layer. Chill overnight.

Serve chilled with your favorite whipped topping and chocolate shavings.

This is a delicious dessert that always surprises people when they find out that it's dairy-free. It's creamy and full of flavor, but not too dense or heavy. Perfect for any special occasion!

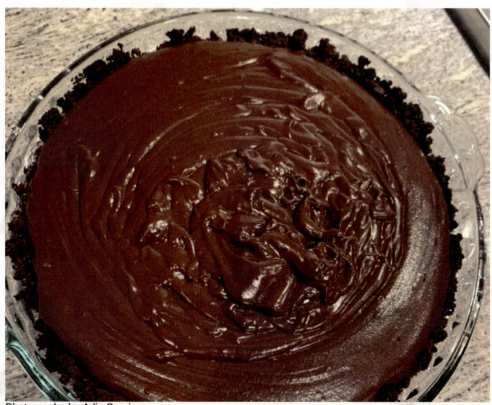

Photography by Adin Services

Sweet Potato Pie

2	Organic Egg Whites
3	Organic Sweet Potatoes
1/4 C	Organic Margarine
2	Organic Egg Yolks
1 C	Organic Palm Sugar
1/4 tsp	Sea Salt
1 tsp	Organic Ground Cinnamon
1/2 tsp	Organic Ground Nutmeg
1/2 tsp	Organic Ground Ginger
1/2 C	Organic Dairy Free Milk

Bake your sweet potatoes wrapped in foil at 400-degrees for 1 to 1 ½ hours. Turn oven down to 350 degrees when done.

In standing mixer beat egg whites until soft peaks form. Set aside in small bowl. In same bowl, mix the baked sweet potatoes on medium until smashed. Add in the other ingredients and mix until combined on medium speed. Remove from mixing stand and fold egg whites into sweet potato filling by hand. Be careful to only incorporate the whites, don't over mix.

Pour pie filling into a prepared pie crust and bake at 350-degrees for 35-40 minutes. Filling will be firm when done.

Graham Cracker Pie Crust – Grain Free

12 – 15   Graham Crackers - Page 180
1/3 C   Organic Margarine

Preheat oven to 300 degrees.

Place graham crackers in baggie and use a rolling pin to crush them into crumbs.

Place margarine in pie dish and place in 300-degree oven, until melted. Remove from oven, add graham crackers and use a fork to combine with the margarine and push into the sides and bottom of pie pan.

When the bottom and sides of the pan are thoroughly covered, place foil over the top of the pie pan (to keep the top from burning) and put back into the oven for 20-25 minutes. You may need more graham cracker crumbs or margarine depending on how large or small you made your graham crackers.

Let cool before filling with your favorite pie filling.

Healthy Nut Fudge – Grain Free

3 oz	100% Organic Dark Chocolate - solid
1/3 C	Organic Coconut Oil
1/3 C	Organic Raw Creamed Honey
1 C	Organic Almond Butter
1 TBSP	Organic Vanilla Extract
Pinch	Pink Himalayan Salt

In stainless steel saucepan place chocolate and coconut oil over low heat until melted. Add honey and combine with chocolate mixture. Add in 1 cup nut butter until smooth and fully incorporated. Take off heat and stir in vanilla extract and salt.

Pour into 8" x 8" pan lined with parchment paper. Take a few tablespoons of almond butter and spoon it on top of the chocolate mixture, then use a knife to cut it into the chocolate and create a pretty pattern.

Place in freezer for 2 hours.

Remove from freezer, lift parchment paper out of pan and place on cutting board. Pull down parchment paper from edges and cut into bite sized cubes. Place in airtight container and refrigerate, separate layers with parchment paper. Keep refrigerated.

This is a healthy, delicious and creamy fudge, suitable for holidays and special occasions, or of course, just because!

You can use varied nut butters to create this fudge, as well as peanut butter, although not considered allergen friendly, it is quite tasty for those who like a peanut butter chocolate combination.

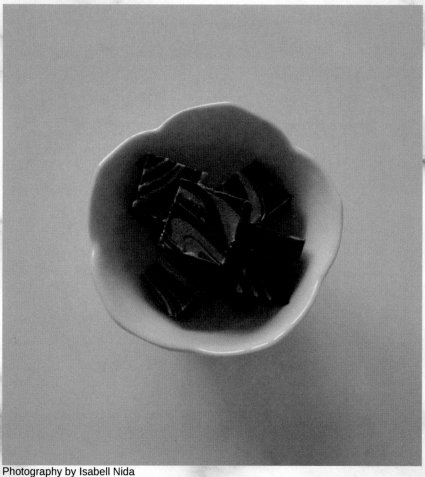

Photography by Isabell Nida

Fudge Topped Brownie Nut Butter Bars

Brownie:

1/4 C	Organic Sorghum Flour
1/4 C	Organic Tapioca Flour
3 TBSP	Organic Cassava Flour
1/4 C	Organic Raw Cocoa Powder
1/4 C	Organic Coconut Palm Sugar
1 tsp	Baking Soda
1/2 tsp	Xanthan Gum
1/2 tsp	Sea Salt
1/2 C	Organic Coconut Oil - melted
1	Organic Egg - beaten
1 tsp	Organic Vanilla Extract
1/4 C	Organic Unsweetened Non-Dairy Milk

Nut Butter Layer:

3/4 C	Organic Nut Butter – your choice
2 TBSP	Organic Raw Creamed Honey
2 tsp	Organic Vanilla Extract
3 TBSP	Organic Coconut Oil

Fudge Topping:

1 TBSP	Organic Coconut Oil
1/2 C	Organic Chocolate Chips
1/2 tsp	Organic Vanilla Extract

Fudge Topped Brownie Nut Butter Bars - continued

Preheat oven to 350 degrees. Use coconut oil to coat an 8" x 8" ceramic or glass dish.

For Brownie, in medium bowl combine, flours, cocoa powder, sugar, baking soda, baking powder and salt. In small bowl, combine egg, vanilla, milk and melted coconut oil. Add wet ingredients to dry and mix well. Spread evenly into prepared dish and put in oven for 20 minutes. Place on wire rack to cool completely.

Once brownie is completely cooled, in a small bowl add all nut butter layer ingredients and mix well. Set aside.

In saucepan on very low heat add coconut oil until melted. Add in chocolate chips and creamed honey until melted and fully combined. Take off heat. Add in vanilla and stir well.

Once all items are prepared, layer the peanut butter on top of the brownie. Then spread the fudge mixture evenly on top. Refrigerate for 3 hours. Cut into bars and serve chilled or at room temperature.

Store in an air-tight container in your refrigerator for up to 5 days.

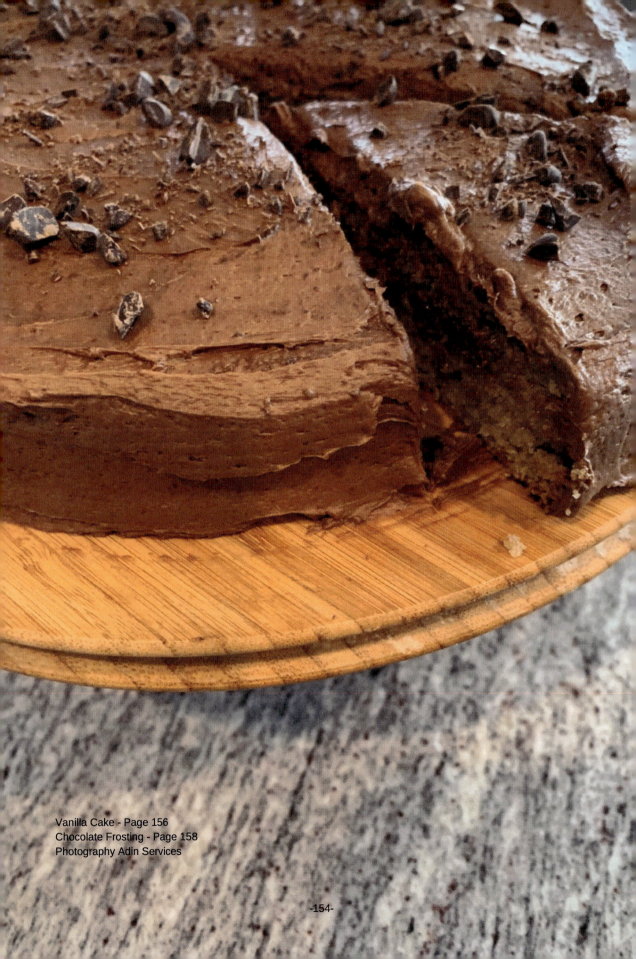

Vanilla Cake - Page 156
Chocolate Frosting - Page 158
Photography Adin Services

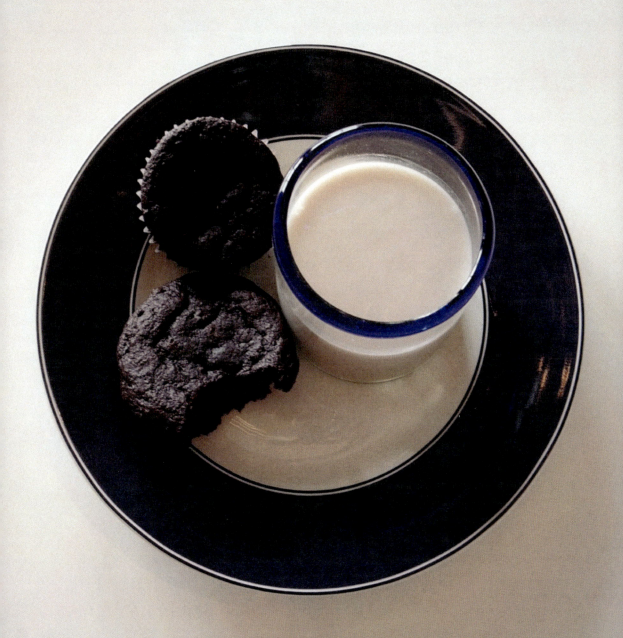

Chocolate Chocolate Chip Cupcakes - Page 160
Photography by Isabell Nida

Vanilla Cake (or Cupcakes) – Grain Free

2 C	Organic Almond Flour
1/4 C	Organic Coconut Flour
1 tsp	Baking Soda
1/2 tsp	Sea Salt
3	Organic Eggs
1/2 C	Organic Maple Syrup
2/3 C	Organic Palm Oil or Coconut Oil - melted
2 tsp	Organic Pure Vanilla Extract

Preheat oven to 350 degrees.

This makes a one-layer cake, or 12 cupcakes. Double the recipe if you want to create a two-layer cake. Line cupcake pan with paper liners or line cake pan bottom with parchment paper and grease sides of pan.

Add all dry ingredients into a large bowl and mix until combined. In a standing mixer add eggs, oil, syrup and extract. Mix thoroughly on medium speed. Once combined add dry ingredients on low speed, slowly. Once combined beat for 30 to 60 seconds on medium speed, scraping sides of bowl often. Place in parchment lined cake pan, or 2/3 full into cupcake liners.

For cake bake for 30-35 minutes at 350 degrees.

Pictured on Page 154 - Photography Adin Services

Vanilla Cake - continued

If making cupcakes bake for 20-25 minutes. Check with a toothpick that your cupcakes are thoroughly cooked before removing from oven. Place on cooling rack for 20 minutes before removing from pan.

You can easily add ½ a cup of your favorite dried fruit or chocolate chips to vary the recipe. Be creative and have fun with it!

This is the perfect cake for a birthday celebration!

Chocolate Frosting

1/2 C	Organic Coconut Palm Sugar
1 1/2 TBSP	Organic Arrowroot Flour
2/3 C	Organic Palm Shortening - not coconut oil
1 tsp	Organic Vanilla Extract
3 TBSP	Organic Raw Cocoa Powder
1-2 TBSP	Organic Unsweetened Dairy-Free Milk

In a blender or food processor mix coconut palm sugar on high until the granules become powdery. This step is very important, don't skip it.

In the mixing bowl of your standing mixer, add powdered coconut palm sugar, arrowroot flour and cocoa powder and combine on slow speed. Add in palm shortening and vanilla extract. If you substitute with coconut oil, the frosting will be runny and greasy. Turn mixer on low and combine, then turn to medium and very slowly add in the milk, until you get the icing to a spreadable but not runny consistency. Once you have it thin enough, turn mixer on high and let it run for a minute, scraping sides of the bowl often.

This is enough frosting to cover a one-layer cake or 12 cupcakes. Double the recipe if you're making a double layer cake.

Pictured on Page 154 - Photography Adin Services

Chocolate Frosting - continued

I sprinkle chopped up unsweetened chocolate on top of the icing to make a better presentation. Or you can sprinkle unsweetened coconut flakes, nuts, or dried fruit.

Be creative, you really can't go wrong.

Chocolate Chocolate-Chip Cupcakes

This is great to make with your kids, no standing mixer is needed and it comes together quickly.

3/4 C	Gluten Free Flour Mix – Page 123
1/2 C	Organic Raw Cocoa Powder
3/4 C	Organic Coconut Palm Sugar
1/2 tsp	Baking Soda
1/2 tsp	Xanthan Gum
3/4 tsp	Baking Powder
1/2 tsp	Sea Salt
1/4 C	Organic Avocado Oil
2	Organic Eggs
3/4 C	Purified Water*
1/3 C	Organic Applesauce
1 tsp	Organic Vanilla Extract
1/2 C	Organic Chocolate Chips

Preheat oven to 350 degrees. Fill cupcake tin with paper liners, set aside.

In large mixing bowl add first seven ingredients from flour mix to salt. Stir well to combine, leaving a well in the center.

In medium mixing bowl, whisk eggs with oil, water, applesauce and extract. Add to dry ingredients and mix

Pictured on Page 155 - Photography by Isabell Nida

Chocolate Chocolate-Chip Cupcakes - continued

well. Fold in chocolate chips.

Place batter into paper lined cupcake pan approximately 2/3 – 3/4 full per liner. Place in pre-heated oven on middle rack for 18-20 minutes. You can test with a cake tester or toothpick to ensure they're thoroughly cooked. Cool on wire rack.

*For variety use strong organic coffee instead of water.

Boston Crème Pie – Grain Free

Custard Ingredients:

1/2 C	Organic Coconut Crème -canned
2 TBSP	Organic Maple Syrup or Creamed Honey
1/4 C	Organic Unsweetened Non-Dairy Milk
1	Organic Egg Yolk
1 tsp	Organic Vanilla Extract

Cake Ingredients:

2 C	Organic Almond Flour
1/4 C	Organic Coconut Flour
1 tsp	Baking Soda
1/2 tsp	Sea Salt
3	Organic Eggs
1/2 C	Organic Maple Syrup
2/3 C	Organic Palm Oil or Coconut Oil
1 tsp	Organic Vanilla Extract

Ganache Ingredients:

1 oz	Organic 100% Dark Chocolate - solid
1/4 C	Organic Coconut Crème
2 TBSP	Organic Palm or Coconut Oil
1/2 tsp	Organic Pure Vanilla Extract
1 TBSP	Organic Raw Creamed Honey

Pictured on Page 145 - Photograpy Adin Services

Boston Crème Pie – continued

Preheat oven at 350 degrees.

Prepare the custard first, as it will need time to cool. In a saucepan add coconut crème and non-dairy milk with syrup and heat over low heat. Once heated slightly add beaten egg yolk and whisk while continuing to heat. This will make the custard thicken, but not like a pudding, it's very gradual and subtle. Once you see it start to thicken, take off heat and add in the vanilla, stir well. Place in glass container in the refrigerator. It will thicken as it cools.

Prepare the Cake. Add all the dry ingredients into a large mixing bowl and combine. In standing mixer add in eggs, oil, syrup and extract and combine on medium speed. Once combined add dry ingredients slowly on low speed, then beat for 30 to 60 seconds on medium speed, make sure to scrape the sides of the bowl a few times. Put batter into greased round cake pan that is lined with parchment paper.

Bake for 35 minutes at 350 degrees. Cool on wire rack for 20 minutes, then place plate on bottom of pan and flip over. It should easily release with parchment paper lining. Remove lining and leave to cool completely (or overnight).

Boston Crème Pie – continued

When you're ready to assemble the cake, cut the cake in half horizontally, to make two layers. The cake must be cool in order to do this successfully. I suggest using a knife that is longer than the cake is wide. This can easily be accomplished with a long bread knife.

Prepare the ganache by placing all ingredients in a small saucepan on low heat. Lightly whisk as the ingredients melt and combine. Once completely melted, take off of heat and set aside to cool.

Put all of the custard on top of the bottom layer of the cake in the center and spread it evenly to the edges.Place the top layer of cake back onto the top of the custard topped layer and adjust so that it is centered on the bottom layer. Pour the cooled ganache very slowly over the top of the cake. Make sure it drips slightly down the edges, but not too much, making sure to cover the entire top of the cake. You can put a few berries on top to garnish or a mint leaf or leave it just as it is.

This makes a beautiful buttery flavored cake with a great presentation. This is definitely a crowd pleaser!

Pineapple Upside Down Cake – Grain Free

Topping:
1/2 C   Organic Coconut Palm Sugar
2 TBSP   Organic Coconut Oil
           Organic Fresh Pineapple Slices & Cherries*

Cake Ingredients:
2 C   Organic Almond Flour
1/4 C   Organic Coconut Flour
1 tsp   Baking Soda
1/2 tsp   Sea Salt
3   Organic Eggs
1/2 C   Organic Maple Syrup or Creamed Honey
2/3 C   Organic Palm Oil or Coconut Oil
2 tsp   Organic Pure Vanilla Extract

Preheat oven to 350 degrees.

In a round (8-9") cake pan, add the coconut palm sugar and coconut oil and place in the middle rack of oven while it preheats to melt the oil - about 15 minutes. Remove from oven and use a spoon to combine and evenly distribute the sugar oil mixture into the bottom of the pan. Add your sliced pineapple and cherries in whatever pattern you like and set pan aside.

Pictured Page 167 - Photography by Adin Services

Pineapple Upside Down Cake – continued

For the cake, add all dry ingredients to large mixing bowl and combine. In standing mixer add in eggs, oil, syrup and extract and combine. Once combined add dry ingredients slowly on low speed. Once combined you can beat for 30 to 60 seconds on medium, scraping the sides of the bowl often. Pour on top of pineapple and sugar topping in prepared cake pan.

Bake for 35 minutes at 350 degrees. When baked, place cake still in the pan on a cooling rack for 20 minutes, then scrape sides of cake and place a plate on the bottom of pan and flip it over. It should easily release and show off the cute design made with the pineapple and cherries.

This is very easy to make and people always assume it's difficult to do. It's a very tasty dessert and no one needs to know it's this simple to make! Keep in refrigerator for up to five days – if it lasts that long! You can serve this warm right after flipping it over.

*I have used frozen cherries before that I've heated up in the microwave and drained off the excess liquid. I have not used, nor do I suggest, canned pineapple for this recipe.

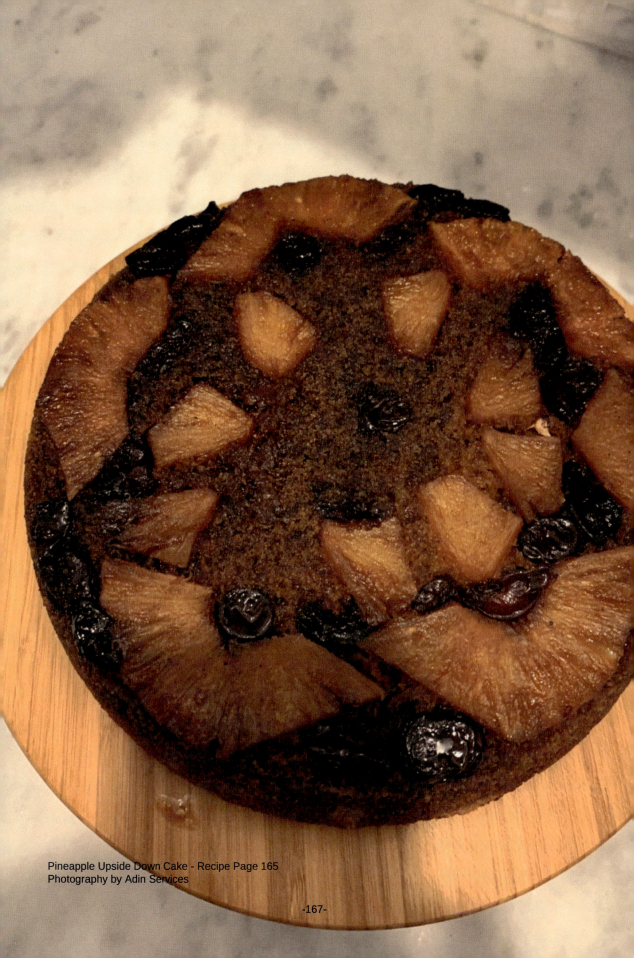

Pineapple Upside Down Cake - Recipe Page 165
Photography by Adin Services

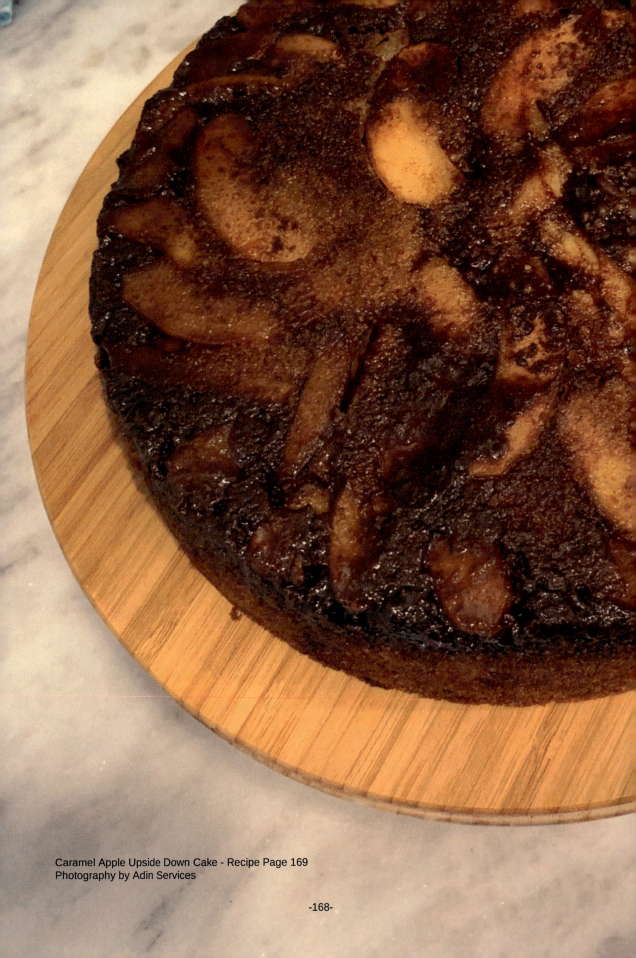

Caramel Apple Upside Down Cake - Recipe Page 169
Photography by Adin Services

Caramel Apple Upside Down Cake – Grain Free

Topping:
1/2 C	Organic Coconut Palm Sugar
2 TBSP	Organic Coconut Oil
1 TBSP	Organic Ground Cinnamon
3	Organic Apples – peeled, cored and sliced

Cake Ingredients:
2 C	Organic Almond Flour
1/4 C	Organic Coconut Flour
1 tsp	Baking Soda
1/2 tsp	Sea Salt
1/2 TBSP	Organic Ground Cinnamon
1/8 tsp	Organic Ground Nutmeg
3	Organic Eggs
1/2 C	Organic Maple Syrup or Creamed Honey
2/3 C	Organic Palm Oil or Coconut Oil
2 tsp	Organic Pure Vanilla Extract

Preheat oven to 350 degrees.

In a round (8-9") cake pan, add the coconut palm sugar, cinnamon and coconut oil and place in the middle rack of oven while it preheats to melt the oil. Leave in oven for 15 minutes. Remove from oven and use a spoon to combine and evenly distribute the sugar oil mixture into

Pictured on Page 168 - Photography Adin Services

Caramel Apple Upside Down Cake – continued

the bottom of the pan. Add your sliced apples in whatever pattern you like and set pan aside.

For the cake, add all dry ingredients in large mixing bowl and combine. In standing mixer add in eggs, oil, syrup and extract and combine. Once combined add dry ingredients slowly on low speed. Once combined beat for 30 to 60 seconds on medium, scraping sides of bowl often. Pour on top of prepared apple topping in cake pan.

Bake for 35 minutes at 350 degrees. Once out of oven, put on cooling rack for 20 minutes, then scrape sides of cake and place a plate on the bottom of pan and flip it over. It should easily release and show off the cute design you made with the apples.

This is very easy to make and people always assume it's difficult to do. It's a very tasty dessert and no one needs to know it's so simple! Keep in refrigerator for up to five days – if it lasts that long! You can serve this warm right after flipping it over.

Apple Crisp – Grain Free

5	Organic Apples - peeled & chopped
1/2 C	Organic Raisins or Dried Cranberries
1 TBSP	Organic Lemon Juice
2 TBSP	Organic Raw Honey
1 TBSP	Organic Cassava Flour
1/2 C	Organic Almond Flour
2 TBSP	Organic Coconut Flour
1/2 C	Organic Coconut Palm Sugar
2 tsp	Organic Ground Cinnamon
1/2 C	Chopped Pecans or Walnuts
1/2 C	Organic Coconut Oil

Pre-heat oven at 350 degrees.

Place apples, raisins, lemon juice, honey and cassava flour in a mixing bowl, stirring to ensure the apples are coated. Place in the bottom of a 9" x 9" baking dish.

In a medium mixing bowl combine flours, sugar, nuts, oil and cinnamon with a pastry blender (or two knives, using a scissor motion) until combined and crumbly. Evenly distribute on top of the apple mixture and place in pre-heated oven for 30-35 minutes.

Apple Cobbler

4	Large Organic Apples
1 TBSP	Organic Lemon Juice
1/3 C	Organic Coconut Palm Sugar
1 TBSP	Organic Ground Cinnamon
1/4 tsp	Organic Ground Nutmeg
1 C	Gluten Free Flour Mix – Page 107
1/2 TBSP	Baking Powder
1/3 C	Organic Margarine or Palm Shortening
1/3 C	Organic Unsweetened Dairy-Free Milk
1/4 tsp	Sea Salt

Preheat oven to 350 degrees.

Peel, core and cut apples into 1" chunks and place in mixing bowl. Add lemon juice and coat apple chunks.

In small bowl combine coconut palm sugar and spices, sprinkle on prepared apple chunks, using spatula to stir to coat. Place in 8" x 8" baking dish and set aside.

In large mixing bowl, combine flour mix, baking soda and salt. Use a pastry cutter (or two butter knives) to cut in margarine or shortening. Once the texture is crumbly and no large chunks are left, add milk and combine until wet, not doughy. Place on top of apples in clumps, evenly distributed. Bake at 350 degrees for 35 minutes. Serve hot or cold.

Cookies

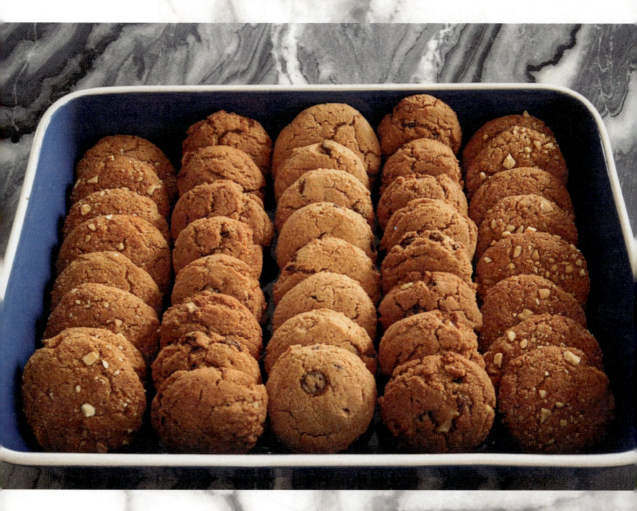

Peanut Butter (outside), Raisin Walnut (2nd & 4th row) & Chocolate Chip Cookies (middle) - Photography by Isabell Nida

Raisin Walnut Cookies – Grain Free

1 C	Organic Almond Flour
1/4 C	Organic Coconut Flour
1/2 TBSP	Organic Ground Cinnamon
1 tsp	Baking Soda
1/2 tsp	Sea Salt
2/3 C	Organic Coconut Palm Sugar
1/3 C	Organic Palm Shortening
1/3 C	Organic Almond Butter
1 tsp	Organic Pure Vanilla Extract
1	Organic Large Egg
1/2 C	Organic Raisins
1/4 C	Walnuts - chopped

Preheat oven to 350 degrees.

Combine all dry ingredients into medium sized bowl, set aside. In standing mixer add coconut palm sugar, palm shortening and almond butter. Combine on low speed. Add in egg and extract and combine until smooth, you might have to scrape the sides of the bowl to ensure its completely combined. Add in dry ingredients until combined thoroughly. Add in raisins and walnuts on lowest speed for thirty seconds.

Pictured Page 173 - Photography by Isabell Nida

Raisin Walnut Cookies - continued

On parchment paper lined baking sheets use a cookie scooper (1") and scoop dough onto cookie sheet, placing 2" apart. I usually put nine cookies on one sheet. Pat the cookie down slightly, not squishing but making sure it doesn't stay in ball form.

Bake for 12 - 14 minutes in pre-heated oven. Take out and leave on sheet for 3 minutes before transferring to cooling racks.

Makes 18 – 20 cookies. Keep in airtight container for up to one week.

Chocolate Chip Cookies – Grain Free

1 C	Organic Almond Flour
1/4 C	Organic Coconut Flour
1 tsp	Baking Soda
1/2 tsp	Sea Salt
1/3 C	Organic Palm Shortening
2/3 C	Organic Coconut Palm Sugar
1/3 C	Organic Almond Butter
1 tsp	Organic Vanilla Extract
1	Organic Large Egg
1/2 C	Organic Chocolate Chips

Preheat oven to 350 degrees.

In mixing bowl, combine dry ingredients from almond flour to salt.

In a standing mixer on medium speed, combine shortening, sugar, almond butter, vanilla and egg until combined. Add in dry ingredients slowly, until combined thoroughly. Lower speed on mixer to low and add in chocolate chips.

On parchment lined baking sheets, use 1" scooper to scoop dough onto parchment paper, placing about 2" apart.

Pictured Page 173 - Photography by Isabell Nida

Chocolate Chip Cookies - continued

Press with the palm of your hand to slightly flatten dough.

Bake for 12-14 minutes, depending on how crispy you'd like your cookies. Cool cookies on wire rack before serving. Makes approximately 18 – 20 cookies.

Date Bars

Cookie:

1 C	Organic Coconut Palm Sugar
1 C	Organic Sorghum Flour
1/2 C	Organic Brown Rice
1/2 C	Organic Arrowroot Flour
1/2 C	Organic Cassava Flour
1/2 tsp	Sea Salt
1/2 tsp	Baking Soda
1 tsp	Xanthan Gum
2/3 C	Organic Coconut Oil

Filling:

2 C	Organic Pitted Organic Dates – chopped
1/2 C	Organic Coconut Palm Sugar
1/4 C	Organic Lemon Juice
1/2 C	Walnuts – chopped

Preheat oven to 350 degrees.

In standing mixer, mix all cookie ingredients on medium until thoroughly combined. Mix may be crumbly.

In saucepan on medium heat add all filling ingredients except walnuts. While heating, stir often, leave on heat until mixture becomes thick like a paste. Remove from heat and add walnuts to the mixture.

Date Bars - continued

In a 10" x 8" greased pan, place half of the cookie mixture on the bottom, pressing and ensuring it's evenly spread. Add the filling and smooth over bottom layer until even. Then place the rest of the cookie layer over the top.

Bake in pre-heated oven for 25-30 minutes. Leave in pan to cool completely. Cut into bars and serve.

Honey Cinnamon Graham Crackers – Grain Free

1 C	Organic Almond Flour
1/4 C	Organic Coconut Flour
1 tsp	Baking Soda
1 tsp	Organic Cinnamon
1/2 tsp	Sea Salt
1/4 C	Organic Creamed Honey
1/2 C	Organic Coconut Palm Sugar
1/3 C	Organic Almond Butter
1 tsp	Organic Vanilla Extract
1	Organic Egg
1/3 C	Organic Palm Shortening

Preheat oven to 275 degrees.

In mixing bowl, combine all dry ingredients, set aside. In standing mixer combine sugars and all wet ingredients on medium speed. Add dry ingredients on low speed and move to medium speed once combined. Beat for one minute, scraping sides often.

Place dough on non-stick cookie sheet or cover regular cookie sheet with parchment paper. Cover with wax paper or parchment paper and roll out the dough. Don't worry if it's not perfectly symmetrical.

Honey Cinnamon Graham Crackers - continued

Use cutter/embosser tool to make rectangular lines in dough. If you don't have one, no worries, it will still work great.

Bake at 275 degrees for 30-40 minutes, making sure the underside of the graham crackers do not burn.

Cool in pan. When cool, cut with a sharp knife over the lines you made (if you didn't make lines, just cut into rectangles or squares). Works great for a graham cracker pie crust - recipe on page 149.

Peanut Butter Cookies – Grain Free

1/3 C	Organic Coconut Oil
3/4 C	Organic Raw Creamed Honey
1/2 C	Coconut Palm Sugar
1/3 C	Organic Peanut Butter
1 tsp	Organic Vanilla Extract
1	Organic Egg
1 C	Organic Almond Flour
3/4 C	Organic Coconut Flour
1 TBSP	Organic Flax Meal
1 tsp	Baking Soda
1/2 tsp	Sea Salt
1 1/2 oz	Organic Peanuts - chopped
1 1/2 TBSP	Organic Coconut Palm Sugar

Preheat oven to 350 degrees, line large cookie sheet with parchment paper.

In standing mixer combine coconut oil, sugar and honey on low setting. Add in peanut butter, vanilla and egg, one at a time and mix each until well combined.

In separate medium mixing bowl, stir together the almond flour, coconut flour, flax meal, salt and baking soda. Add dry ingredients to wet in standing mixer and combine well.

Pictured Page 173 - Photography by Isabell Nida

Peanut Butter Cookies - continued

Combine chopped peanuts and coconut palm sugar in small bowl.

Using a 1" metal scooper, scoop out 1" balls of dough (or use your hands if you don't have a scooper) coat dough in the chopped peanut and sugar mixture, place on cookie sheet. Use the palm of your hand to flatten the balls slightly.

Bake for 12 - 14 minutes. Leave on pan for 3 minutes after removing from oven, then transfer to wire cooling racks.

Makes 18 – 20 Cookies.

You can easily make these almond butter cookies, by substituting peanut butter with almond butter and chopped peanuts with chopped almonds. It's delicious either way.

Chocolate - Chocolate Chip Cookies – Grain Free

1 C	Organic Almond Flour
1/4 C	Organic Coconut Flour
1 tsp	Baking Soda
1/2 tsp	Sea Salt
3 TBSP	Organic Cocoa Powder Unsweetened
1/3 C	Organic Palm Shortening
3/4 C	Organic Coconut Palm Sugar
1/3 C	Organic Almond Butter
1 tsp	Organic Vanilla Extract
1	Organic Large Egg
1/2 C	Organic Chocolate Chips

Preheat oven to 350 degrees.

In mixing bowl, combine dry ingredients from almond flour to cocoa powder.

In standing mixer on medium speed, combine shortening, sugar, almond butter, vanilla and egg until combined. Add in dry ingredients slowly, until combined thoroughly. Lower speed on mixer and add in chocolate chips.

Chocolate - Chocolate Chip Cookies - continued

On parchment lined baking sheets, use 1" scooper to scoop dough onto parchment paper. Keeping about 2" apart. Press with the palm of your hand to slightly flatten dough.

Bake for 12-14 minutes, depending on how crispy you'd like your cookies. Cool cookies on wire rack before serving. Makes approximately 18 – 20 cookies.

Pumpkin Spice Cookies – Grain Free

1 C	Organic Almond Flour
1/4 C	Organic Coconut Flour
1 tsp	Baking Soda
1/2 tsp	Sea Salt
1 tsp	Organic Pumpkin Spice Seasoning
1/3 C	Organic Palm Shortening
3/4 C	Organic Coconut Palm Sugar
1/3 C	Organic Almond Butter
1 tsp	Organic Vanilla Extract
1	Organic Egg
1/3 C	Organic Raisins (optional)
3 TBSP	Organic Coconut Palm Sugar
2 tsp	Organic Pumpkin Spice Seasoning

Preheat oven to 350 degrees.

In mixing bowl, combine dry ingredients from almond flour to seasoning.

In a standing mixer on medium speed, combine shortening, sugar, almond butter, vanilla and egg until combined. Add in dry ingredients slowly, until combined thoroughly. Lower speed to low and add in raisins.

Pumpkin Spice Cookies - continued

In small shallow bowl combine sugar and spices. Use 1" scooper to scoop dough and place in bowl with sugar. Coat thoroughly and put on parchment lined baking sheets, keeping about 2" apart. Press with the palm of your hand to slightly flatten dough.

Cook for 12-14 minutes, depending on how crispy you'd like your cookies. Cool cookies on wire rack before serving. Makes approximately 18 – 20 cookies.

Coconut Cookies – Grain Free

1 C	Organic Almond Flour
1/4 C	Organic Coconut Flour
1 TBSP	Organic Flax Seed Meal
1 tsp	Baking Soda
1/2 tsp	Sea Salt
1/3 C	Organic Coconut Oil
1/4 C	Organic Raw Creamed Honey
1/3 C	Organic Coconut Palm Sugar
1/3 C	Organic Coconut Butter
1	Organic Egg
1 tsp	Organic Vanilla Extract
1/2 C	Organic Flaked Unsweetened Coconut
1 1/2 tsp	Organic Coconut Palm Sugar

Preheat oven to 350 degrees.

In mixing bowl combine all dry ingredients.

In standing mixer, combine oil, honey, sugar, butter, egg and extract on medium speed. Add dry ingredients slowly until thoroughly combined.

In shallow bowl combine the flaked coconut and palm sugar. Using a 1" scooper scoop dough into bowl with flaked coconut.

Coconut Cookies - continued

Roll dough in coconut and place on baking sheets lined with parchment paper. Lightly press the dough down with your palm.

Bake in preheated oven for 12-14 minutes. Cool on wire rack.

Gingerbread Cookies – Grain Free

1 C	Organic Almond Flour
1/4 C	Organic Coconut Flour
1 tsp	Baking Soda
1/2 tsp	Sea Salt
1/2 TBSP	Organic Ground Ginger
1 tsp	Organic Ground Cinnamon
1/2 tsp	Organic Ground Cloves
1/3 C	Organic Palm Shortening
2/3 C	Organic Coconut Palm Sugar
1/3 C	Organic Almond Butter
2 TBSP	Organic Blackstrap Molasses
1 tsp	Organic Vanilla Extract
1	Organic Egg
1/3 C	Organic Raisins - optional

Preheat oven to 350 degrees.

In mixing bowl, combine dry ingredients from almond flour to spices.

In a standing mixer on medium speed, combine shortening, sugar, almond butter, molasses, vanilla and egg. Add in dry ingredients slowly, until combined thoroughly. Lower speed on mixer to low and add in raisins.

Gingerbread Cookies - continued

Use 1" scooper to scoop dough and place on parchment lined baking sheets, keeping about 2" apart. Press with the palm of your hand to slightly flatten dough.

Cook for 12-14 minutes, depending on how crispy you'd like your cookies. Cool cookies on wire rack before serving. Makes approximately 18 – 20 cookies.

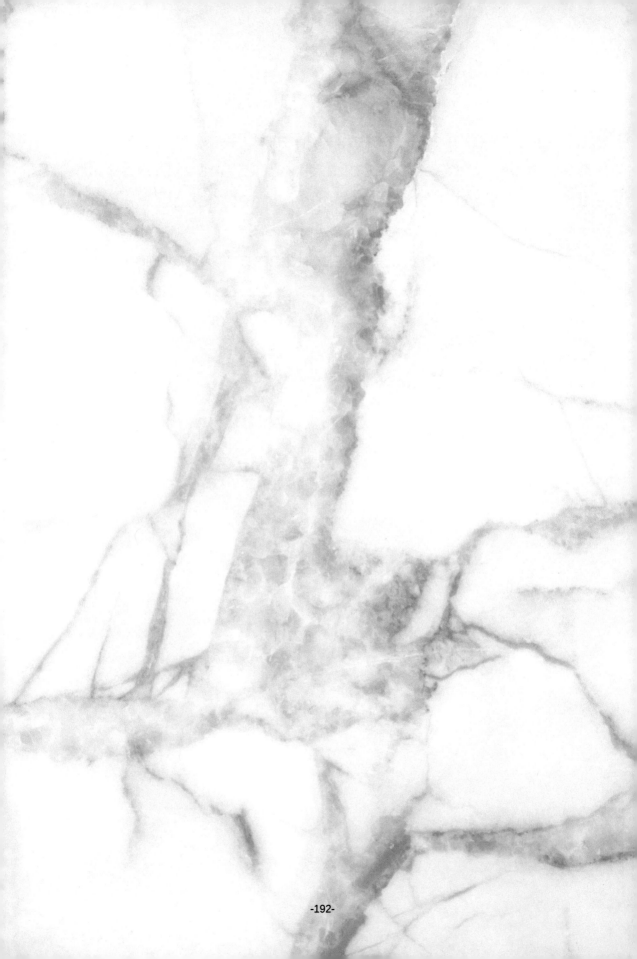

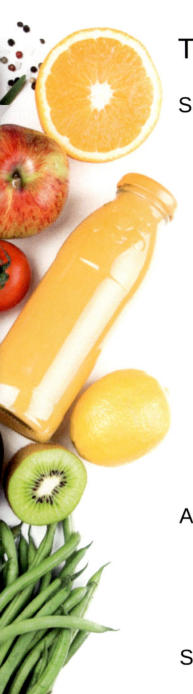

Table of Contents

Sauces, Condiments, Dips & Spices

Ketchup	29
Mayonnaise	30
Tzatziki Sauce	31
Ranch Dressing	32
Thousand Island Dressing	33
Honey Mustard Dressing/Dip	34
Mango Sauce	35
Pineapple Sauce	36
Pizza Sauce	37
B-B-Q Sauce	38
Tartar Sauce	39
Cocktail Sauce	40
Peanut Butter Fruit Dip	41
Cream Cheese Fruit Drip	43
Jerk Spice	44
Mediterranean Spice	45

Appetizers

Scallop Appetizer	47
Buffalo Chicken Wings	49
Caribbean Jerk Chicken Wings	51
Guacamole	52

Salads

Chicken Salad	54
Baked Potato Salad	55
Sweet Potato Salad	57
Grilled Romaine Salad	58
Waldorf Salad	59

Sides

Home Made French Fries	61
Scalloped Potatoes	62
Sweet Potato Fries	64
Sweet Potato Hash	66
Sweet Potato Casserole	67
Mashed Cauliflower	69
Roasted Broccolini	70
Spiraled Vegetables	71
Sauteed Mushrooms & Onions	72
Green Bean Casserole	73
Creamy Salsa Rice	74
Chicken Fried Rice	75
Thanksgiving Day Stuffing	77

Entrée's

Summer Marinated Chicken	80
Mediterranean Chicken	81
Chicken and Apples	83
Creamy Chicken and Artichokes	85
Sauced Salmon	86
Seared Ahi Tuna with Sauce	87
Tuna Casserole	88
Jerk Spiced Mahi-Mahi	91
Island Pineapple Shrimp	92
Crab Cakes	93
Shrimp Tacos	95
Individual Turkey Meatloaves	96
B-B-Q Meatloaf	98
Baked Ziti	99
Stewed Flat Iron Steaks	101
Meatballs	103
Perfectly Grilled Steak	104

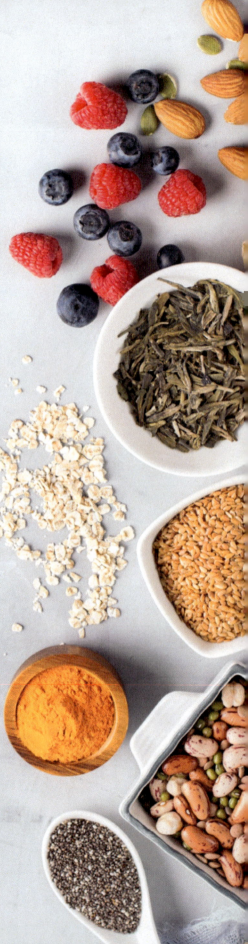

Soups

Chicken Noodle Soup	106
Creamy Shrimp Chowder	107
Creamy Tomato Dill Soup	108
Italian Beef Soup	109

Breakfast

Pancake Mix	111
Healthy Eggs Benedict	112
French Toast	114
Hash Browns	115
Cream Cheese Breakfast Danish	117

Breads

Gluten-Free Sourdough Starter	121
Gluten-Free Bread Mix	123
Sourdough Bread	125
Fluffy Sandwich Bread	128
Raisin Bread	130
Flat Bread	133
Apple Cinnamon Muffins	134
Orange Cranberry Bread	136
Pizza Dough	138

Smoothies

Cherry Smoothie	141
Chocolate Cherry Smoothie	142
Banana Nut Smoothie	142
Pina Colada Smoothie	143
Berry Smoothie	143
Chocolate Nut Butter Chia Smoothie	144

Desserts

Chocolate Silk Pie	146
Sweet Potato Pie	148
Graham Cracker Pie Crust	149
Healthy Nut Fudge	150
Fudge Topped Peanut Butter Brownie Bars	152
Vanilla Cake	156
Vanilla Cupcakes	156
Chocolate Frosting	158
Chocolate Chocolate-Chip Cupcakes	160
Boston Crème Pie	162
Pineapple Upside Down Cake	165
Caramel Apple Upside Down Cake	169
Apple Crisp	171
Apple Cobbler	172

Cookies

Raisin Walnut Cookies	174
Chocolate Chip Cookies	176
Date Bars	178
Honey Cinnamon Graham Crackers	180
Peanut Butter Cookies	182
Chocolate Chocolate-Chip Cookies	184
Pumpkin Spice Cookies	186
Coconut Cookies	188
Gingerbread Cookies	190

Don't wait for illness to start valuing wellness
— unknown

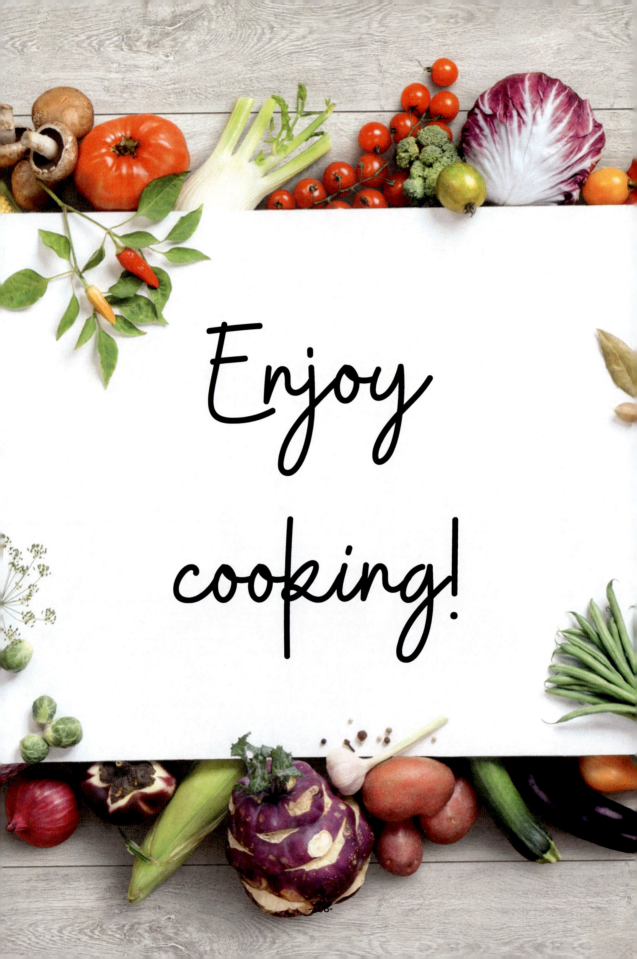

Follow the Author at:

Author's Website
www.hlnidaauthor.com

on Amazon
www.amazon.com/H.L.-Nida

on Goodreads
www.goodreads.com/author/H_L_Nida

Check out my Romance Novel Series as well!

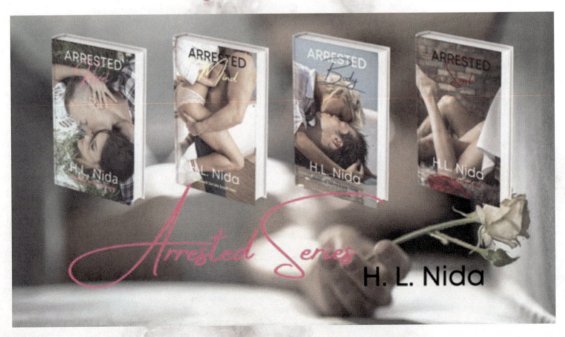